TRAIN YOUR BRAIN TO **Get Thin**

TRAIN YOUR BRAIN TO Get Thin

PRIME YOUR GRAY CELLS FOR

WEIGHT LOSS, WELLNESS, AND EXERCISE

Melinda Boyd, MPH, MHR, RD with Michele Noonan, PhD

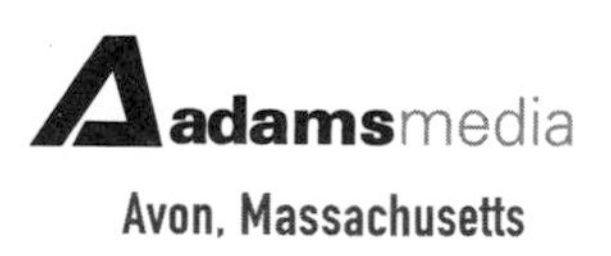

Avon, Massachusetts

Published by
Adams Media, a division of F+W Media, Inc.
57 Littlefield Street, Avon, MA 02322. U.S.A.
www.adamsmedia.com

Contains material adapted and abridged from *365 Ways to Boost Your Metabolism* by Rachel Laferriere, MS, RD, copyright © 2010 by F+W Media, Inc., ISBN 10: 1-4405-0213-7, ISBN 13: 978-1-4405-0213-2; and *Train Your Brain to Get Rich* by Teresa Aubele, PhD, Douglas K. Freeman, JD, LLM, Lee Hauser, PhD, and Susan Reynolds, copyright © 2011 by F+W Media, Inc., ISBN 10: 1-4405-2808-X, ISBN 13: 978-1-4405-2808-8.

ISBN 10: 1-4405-4015-2
ISBN 13: 978-1-4405-4015-8
eISBN 10: 1-4405-4362-3
eISBN 13: 978-1-4405-4362-3

Printed in the United States of America.

10 9 8 7 6 5 4 3 2 1

The information in this book should not be used for diagnosing or treating any health problem. You should always consult a trained medical professional before starting a health program, taking any form of medication, or embarking on any fitness program. The author and publisher disclaim any liability arising directly or indirectly from the use of this book.

This publication is designed to provide accurate and authoritative information with regard to the subject matter covered. It is sold with the understanding that the publisher is not engaged in rendering legal, accounting, or other professional advice. If legal advice or other expert assistance is required, the services of a competent professional person should be sought.

—From a *Declaration of Principles* jointly adopted by a Committee of the American Bar Association and a Committee of Publishers and Associations

Many of the designations used by manufacturers and sellers to distinguish their product are claimed as trademarks. Where those designations appear in this book and Adams Media was aware of a trademark claim, the designations have been printed with initial capital letters.

This book is available at quantity discounts for bulk purchases.
For information, please call 1-800-289-0963.

CONTENTS

INTRODUCTION

"Our greatest battles are that with our own minds."

—Jameson Frank

Jameson Frank was right—your battle to be thin starts with your mind. If you're someone who has spent years struggling to manage your weight, yo-yo dieting and never the getting long-term results you desire, *Train Your Brain to Get Thin* is just the book you need to give you the knowledge and confidence to get started down the right path to a new, thin, and healthy you.

The brain has remained a mystery for years, but recent advances have led to a better understanding of its complexities. We now know that understanding the key functions of the brain allows you to have better control over your own destiny and that the brain can, in fact, change in positive ways to better reach desired outcomes, like losing unwanted excess body fat. The brain is ever changing, just like the shape of your body, so why not harness the power of your mind to help you shed the pounds and keep them off once and for all?

Train Your Brain to Get Thin combines recent breakthroughs in neuroscience with weight loss principles to help you learn how to:

- *Understand the complicated mechanisms of your brain*—how it works for and against you in your quest to get thin.
- *Lose more weight*, by strengthening the thoughtful, analytic part of your brain so you can identify past weight loss pitfalls and learn how to eat and live right to keep yourself thin.
- *Stay on track to get your look-good, feel-good body*, by short-circuiting harmful habits that result in flawed reasoning.

- *Rebound from weight loss setbacks*, without getting caught up by your brain's fight-or-flight response.
- *Make lifelong changes to benefit your health and your waistline*, by taking full advantage of your brain when setting goals.
- *Achieve desired weight loss goals*, by strengthening the brain's ability to tune out distractions and remain focused on the task at hand.

All those tools and more will help you start the process of training your brain to get your weight under control. If you want to use your body's most valuable asset to take control over the way you look and feel about yourself, don't waste another minute . . . your thin body awaits!

CHAPTER 1

WHAT IS THIN?

It's easy to close your eyes and think of what you look like thin. Maybe it was how you looked a few years back. Perhaps this image is how you'd always hoped that your body would look like with a little less weight. Thin is the image you wish to present to others; however, there is more to this. We use the word *thin* because it sounds good. We think of it as something positive. In this book, the word *thin* is used to describe a weight where you are not only healthy, but feel good about yourself as well. This doesn't mean super skinny (which is just as unhealthy as obesity), and this doesn't mean forcing your body to get to a weight you used to be when you were in high school or college. The key is not to focus on achieving an unrealistic weight. Understanding what it means to be thin means letting go of images of movie stars and runway models. It means embracing who you are and understanding that everyone has a different body. You have to work with what you have, not against it, and find the weight that's right for you. A weight that reduces disease risk, but lets you feel comfortable. Having an unrealistic perception of what thin means to—and for—you will hold you back on your quest to shed those unwanted pounds.

You may not be aware of this, but much of what you know about weight, weight loss, and your thoughts about diets has already been ingrained in your brain. This knowledge resulted from what your parents looked like and what they did over the years to lose, gain, or maintain their weight. In order to train your brain to get thin, you need to know what information is tucked away in your memory and how the way your brain comprehends diet habits could have more of an effect than you realize.

In this chapter, you'll learn how to look deep into your mind/brain to see just how much it does (or doesn't!) know about nutrition and healthy lifestyles. We'll discuss the concept of weight loss at a basic level, how your brain understands this, and how the ideas you may have about weight loss may be affecting your ability to lose weight without you even realizing it. Now, before you jump right into learning about your brain and the way it thinks about weight loss, let's spend a few minutes assessing your need to train your brain to get thin.

WHY YOU NEED TO TRAIN YOUR BRAIN TO GET THIN

Chances are you're not 100 percent comfortable at your weight and aren't living a healthy life, and unless you are already at that stage, you're probably not maximizing your brain to work at its peak capacity in losing weight and keeping it off. Let's start off by determining where you weigh in on the get thin scale.

The *How I'm Doing on the Weight Management Front* Quiz

1. **When it came to food, my parents:**

   A. taught me how to enjoy a variety of foods, especially fruits and vegetables.

   B. generally set a good example, but didn't talk much about foods and health.

   C. cooked some meals at home, but didn't teach us about portion sizes when eating out.

   D. fed us everything and anything without paying attention to what was in the food.

2. When it came to managing weight, my parents:

A. shared the importance of a healthy diet to keep weight in check.

B. went through phases where they worked to change their diet to meet healthy guidelines.

C. usually followed the latest diet craze.

D. didn't express a concern over managing their weight.

3. When it comes to my weight loss habits, in the past:

A. I have tried to make healthy food choices and exercise when I have the time.

B. I have tried to make permanent changes to my diet, but they never seemed to last.

C. I tried what everyone else was trying, lost a little weight, but always gained it back.

D. I have been hopping from fad diet to fad diet.

4. Once I decide I want to lose weight, I:

A. make a plan and get focused.

B. think about where I can make changes in my eating habits, but often forget about exercising.

C. think about what reward I want to give myself when I lose the weight.

D. skip meals.

5. When it comes to making food choices, I:

A. think about the benefit the food may provide.

B. give in to my cravings, but try to balance it out during the day with foods I know are healthy.

C. stick with what is convenient or available.

D. put taste before everything else.

6. When making a decision about a food, I:

A. research it by looking at the nutrition information and ingredients.

B. check the labels to make sure I know how much is in a serving.

C. peek at the nutrition information if it's there, but if it isn't readily available I will still eat the food.

D. don't put much thought into what the food contains, how much is a serving, or how many calories it has.

7. I know ______ about nutrition:

A. a good amount.

B. some, but not enough.

C. very little.

D. not a whole lot.

8. Everything I know about weight loss has come from:

A. researching a variety of sources that I trust for weight loss and nutrition information.

B. a combination of research on healthy eating and books on the latest diets.

C. the different diets I have tried over the years.

D. what friends have told me or I have read about in magazines, books, and on the Internet.

Answer Key

If you chose mostly As, you have a strong positive relationship with food and understanding of weight loss to use as a base, but you could use a boost to push you out of your rut. Your brain is in a prime position for training and will respond in a positive manner to the tips offered throughout this book. In no time, you'll be on your way to getting thin—and being happy.

If you chose mostly Bs, your healthy lifestyle and weight loss knowledge has some of the basics down, but definitely has room to grow positively. With a little work, you can strengthen your weight loss knowledge, learn strategies to help your brain work harder for you, and decrease your weight. This book is packed with lots of great ideas for you to help you reshape your thought patterns and get you to your dream body.

If you chose mostly Cs, there may be a lot of work still to be done, but you're eager to learn and ready to make changes. With a little focused fine-tuning, your brain will soon help you get your body looking and feeling good.

If you chose mostly Ds, your brain has a lot of catching up to do. You simply weren't given the knowledge you needed to keep you at a healthy weight or help you lose the weight to get there. But don't worry, because it's not too late. Changing your approach to weight loss won't be nearly as difficult as you might fear. You can get your brain up and running in no time.

WHY YOUR BRAIN IS WORKING TO GET CAUGHT UP

Thanks to millions of years of evolution, we have developed into very intelligent beings. When it comes to managing weight, however, we are influenced by the body's mechanisms designed to get us through times of famine. This means saving excess weight so we have something to use for energy if a time comes when food is scarce. The only problem is that this doesn't happen the same way it did in ancient times. Today we have developed reliable food sources that provide us with a food supply very different from that of our ancestors. Unfortunately, your brain is still influenced by ancient-brain thinking and may perceive going for periods of time without food (like when you skip meals) as times of famine. As a result of this famine, your brain will slow your metabolism to help you hold on to energy stores for the future. Human society has evolved, but the human brain still has some catching up to do.

Your Brain's Shortcomings

Your brain is top notch when it comes to certain things—like recognizing simple patterns or even providing emotional responses in the blink of an eye—but it does lag behind on other tasks. It is difficult for your brain to understand the complexities of food choices and quickly process all that we have to go through when making food choices in a hurry, which many people are when they haven't planned their meal in advance. The brain receives signals from the stomach in response to the need to eat, but there is the added component of the brain getting the message that we *want* to eat instead of just getting the message when the *need* to eat is present.

Fortunately, we are on the frontier of new brain exploration, and this is dishing up some truly exciting insights into the inner workings of the mind and how you can take full advantage of your brain's potential. Thanks to new discoveries in neuroscience, we all have the potential to comprehend so much more about how this marvelously complex structure works and what we can do to help in its development for all aspects of our lives, including managing our weight.

Throughout the book you'll find lots of ideas, tips, and insights to get you zooming along on your quest to get thin . . . but first you have to establish what thin means to you!

WHAT DOES BEING THIN MEAN TO YOU?

Your immediate thoughts might turn to a specific number on the scale, but in fact there is more to your own *thin*. This is only your weight, and while you may see this number on the scale daily, weekly, or just when you visit the doctor, this is not the complete picture. As you move through the chapters of this book, you will be better able to recognize how you can harness the power of your brain to enrich your understanding of *thin*, thereby achieving happiness in all aspects of your life.

WHY THE NUMBER ON THE SCALE ITSELF DOESN'T MOTIVATE YOUR BRAIN

Your weight by itself doesn't satisfy a basic need for survival, like food or water. It's just a number on the scale, and it can change daily—even hourly—but it's what that number *represents* to us that has value. Your weight is therefore called a "secondary reinforcer" because, while it can be used to classify your weight status, or show that you are at a certain desirable weight, it isn't actually a primary reward. When looking at the scale, your train of thought can often go something like this:

Weight on the scale (secondary reinforcer) → fit into smaller clothes (secondary reinforcer) → attract a suitable mate (secondary reinforcer) → fall in love (secondary reinforcer) → create offspring (primary reward).

Thus, the number on the scale plays a role based on your view of it and how it helps you in other aspects of your life. The problem is that the number on the scale doesn't tell the whole picture, so you are better off taking this as only one measure of thin, and looking to other markers, like energy level and comfort in clothing. Whether it's the number on the scale, your BMI (Body Mass Index), or your clothing size, it seems like there is always a number making its way into your quest for thin. Unfortunately, your brain can have difficulty when there is subjectivity involved. For example, if you have a big dream that is filled with lots of reinforcers, your brain could wind up so overwhelmed that it ends up relying on emotions rather than logic to decide which reinforcer needs to take precedence. Finding out what is at the root of your desires and splitting dreams up into smaller, and therefore more attainable, goals will make it easier on your logical brain to work with you to achieve those goals.

WHAT DOES THE TERM *THIN* MEAN TO YOU?

Maybe you have heard about Body Mass Index. This is a method that doctors and other clinicians use to determine your weight status. While there may be some flaws with this method—for example, it can't differentiate between lean muscle mass and body fat—it is still commonly used and serves as a way to assess your own height and weight in relation to each other (and ultimately against others), in order to determine your risk for developing chronic diseases linked to carrying around excess body weight, such as diabetes and cardiovascular disease. It is important to mention this because you may hear this term from time to time, either from your doctor or in the media.

Your ideal *thin* weight will usually fall within the healthy weight range, which means a weight less than the level determined for overweight status, but more than the category for underweight status (let's call this "skinny," and note that there are health risks associated with this too). There is a big range here to allow you to find a comfortable, *thin* weight, which will help you find the thin that works for you. There are other ways to determine where your healthy weight should be, but for the purposes of training your brain to get thin, you want your *thin* weight to be one that is known to reduce health risks, while also being a weight that your brain perceives as good looking.

So take a minute to really think about what the word *thin* means to you. Forget about the numbers on the scale, forget about clothing sizes. You should know where you feel your best, inside and out. Defining exactly what thin looks like to you and how you value this will be important to your process of losing weight.

Where Did You Get Your Body Image and Weight Ideas?

To understand why you want to be thin or what thin means to you, it is important to think about where you developed your ideas about being thin in the first place. Did these ideas come from your parents? Is your concept of thin rooted in magazines and movies? Do you determine what equals thin based on other members of your peer group? Where you developed your ideas about what thin looks like or how it registers on a scale are dependent upon outside sources, and these impact how you see both yourself and where you want to be, weight-wise.

Consider the kinds of messages you may have received growing up. Did you ever hear the word "skinny" and think of this as a positive descriptor of weight or body shape? Did your mother tell you that only "skinny" people are successful and glamorous? Did your best friend tell you that only "skinny" people are pretty and will meet their Prince Charming? Many times we equate "skinny" with thin, but it's important to think beyond those words. Think of "skinny" as the opposite extreme of "obese," and consider "thin" to be a healthier word to use in regards to body image and how you perceive a slender body shape.

Examine the messages you heard growing up and their effects on you. Challenge these ideas of what someone should look like, so that you can make different decisions about your own healthy weight goal than you may have aimed for in the past. For example, if you are trying to fit into size 0 jeans because you want to be "stick thin"—perhaps you heard growing up that this was a desirable way to look—consider if this was ever the body type you were meant to have and whether getting to that weight is healthy or even realistic. Forcing yourself into a vision of thin that just isn't you may be holding you back from ever being happy at a healthy, and realistic, *thin* weight.

Respond below by completing the blanks in these statements in order to get a feeling for whether your (conscious or unconscious) ideas about weight and body image are holding you back.

1. Thin people get that way because

____

2. Thin people are thin because

____

3. Thin people are able to do

____

4. The relationship between weight and happiness is

____

5. I will always weigh

____

6. I could weigh

____

7. With my current body weight, I do not deserve

____

8. Parents impact their children's weight by

____

9. Never rely on your weight to

____

10. I am afraid to try and get to a healthy weight because

____

Note that questions 6–10 reflect limitation beliefs—beliefs that limit you or hold you back in some way—based on weight status. As you move through this book, you will learn about how these negative thought patterns can significantly interfere with your goal of getting to your healthy weight and staying there.

Do You Have What It Takes to Be Thin?

Everyone has what it takes to be thin, but for some people this comes naturally. For others it takes more work, and for others it is *really* hard work. This all has to do with differences in the human body, but that only accounts for part of the success or failure associated with maintaining a healthy weight. The rest has to do with behaviors and lifestyles, and this has to do with your brain. Sure, knowing about nutrition, what to eat, what not to eat, and how to find a balance is important, but how you apply this knowledge and make lifestyle changes will depend on the training you learn from this book. Those who have successfully lost weight have made changes to their diet and exercise routines rather than making drastic, short-lived adjustments in search of some unattainable weight loss goal. So do you have what it takes to retrain your brain to keep those lifestyle changes in place and get you to your thin body once and for all? Read on, and find out.

IF YOU WANT TO GET THIN, GET HAPPY!

Many people think that being a certain weight or fitting into a certain clothing size will make them happy—even though every person who is thin isn't necessarily happy. Psychologists and researchers alike have demonstrated time and time again that staying positive and being happy leads to better outcomes, more self-confidence, more energy, and, of course, more brainpower. This achievable combination greatly improves your ability of getting to your goal weight and staying there. In fact, when your brain feels optimistic and positively charged, it will operate at a much more effective level than when you have negative feelings or thought patterns.

Focus on Happiness

Research suggests that happiness can influence your choice of a healthy lifestyle and may even help your brain reinforce behaviors regulated by positive emotions, rather than behaviors regulated by negative emotions such as fear, insecurity, or loneliness. Happiness keeps both your brain and your body healthier by lowering levels of stress hormones and inflammation. Besides feeling more relaxed and content, there are plenty of other reasons why it makes a difference to be happy, especially when it comes to your brain's health. Your happiness can:

- Encourage the development of synapses
- Elevate mental efficiency
- Increase your ability to think and analyze
- Affect your perception of your surroundings
- Improve attentiveness

This makes it easy to see why happiness is so important. Happy thought patterns lead to more happy thoughts. When you are happy you can be in better control of the decisions that you make and feel more confident when it comes to healthy behaviors that impact weight.

One study found that people who wrote down three very specific things that truly made them happy each day for a week were actually happier than people who didn't do this daily. Interestingly, this continued to be the trend after one-, three-, and six-month follow-ups, and if you can believe it, even some time after the study was completed. Researchers believe that the people who were focused on those specific three things, the ones that they determined made them truly happy, had basically trained their brains to be on the lookout for other things that resulted in their happiness. Now that you know about this little trick, you can apply this concept to your own quest for thin by looking for three things that you know you have done each day.

IS THIN YOUR DESTINY?

At this time humans are the only species known to have an awareness of our brains and to know that our bodies can adapt as needed, which means that you can undoubtedly train your brain to be successful, to accomplish your life goals, to become the best you, to have the body that you desire, to be healthy and feel energized to enjoy life to its fullest, and so on. This requires that you focus, possess dedication, become accountable for your actions, and utilize persistence; it sounds tough, but, in the end, you *can* train your brain to get you thin.

We'll provide you with the specific actions you can take to help maximize your brain power, giving it some fine tuning that will help it work better for you. You'll be able to balance out your emotions with your rational thinking side when it comes to decision making, and to stimulate your brain to grow and expand, all while working to drop those pounds off your body frame once and for all. So for now, here's the bad news, and of course the good news, when it comes to teaching your brain to transform your body:

The Bad News:

- The evolution of your brain has happened slowly, so as a result it still reverts to ancient, innate responses, which can foil your best efforts at healthy habits from time to time.
- Your brain is already wired to react quickly and instinctively when it senses fear; reflection unfortunately comes later, long after panic has set in.

- Unless you challenge your brain from time to time, it will settle into neuronal ruts and habits.
- Your brain will degenerate: idle synapses will dissolve and no new synapses will form unless you challenge your mind.
- The chemistry of your brain can create unbalanced behavior.
- Both drugs and alcohol can have a severe impact on your brain function.
- Your brain loses certain firepower with the aging process (but gains new abilities).

The Good News:

- Your brain is here to serve you.
- Even a damaged brain has the capability of regenerating.
- Your brain will generate new synapses when fresh activities necessitate them.
- Your brain will strengthen and fortify neuronal pathways already in place, when needed.
- Your brain can be rewired, engaging atypical regions to execute needed tasks.
- You can do things to enhance your brain chemistry; although, if necessary, you can use medication to assist in improving your brain function and help with emotional reactivity.
- Your brain can learn from your mind how to hold back fear.
- You can train your brain to do many things, like concentrate and learn new skills.
- You can do things that will aid your brain in staying agile and healthy.
- Older brains will become wiser brains, so it's really never too late to teach it new tricks.

It's starting to sound pretty good, isn't it? That's because there are so many actions you can take to train your brain to get thin. In this book we'll talk about the many ways you can work daily at getting yourself thin, but first you will need to know all about the basics of your brain and how it works. Turn the page to take the first step on your expedition to a thinner life!

CHAPTER 2

THE INNER WORKINGS OF YOUR BRAIN

Principle: Your splendid brain is at your beck and call.

Without a doubt, your brain is the most complex organ within your body. Its capabilities include processing several modalities of sensory information at lightning speed, and controlling organs, movement, and conscious thought. You can put this powerhouse to work for you each and every day as you whittle away the pounds and develop a healthier lifestyle.

Your highly complex brain:

- Is responsible for monitoring and controlling all body functions including breathing, heartbeat, blood circulation, and even digestion
- Handles your response to any pain or pressure you may feel
- Directs all movement of your muscles
- Experiences and implements all of your many moods
- Handles the complex task of managing your memories
- Connects memories with thoughts to form complex associations
- Executes abstract thinking
- Is responsible for creating and integrating your identity

Pretty amazing, isn't it? Plus, that was just a short rundown of some of the amazing tasks your brain is capable of each day.

Just like any other organ, all the parts of your brain, large or small, will play a role in keeping your brain functioning at its best. Understanding how these parts work together to achieve a healthy, fully functioning, regenerative, and expanding brain gives you the power to use your brain as efficiently as possible, making it into a well-oiled machine that will transform you into a healthy, happy, and thin *you*. While you may have a hard time understanding all of the details the first time you read through this chapter, don't give up. The more you understand, the better you can personalize how you train your brain to get thin!

ARE YOU A WHIZ WHEN IT COMES TO YOUR BRAIN?

So, how much do you really know about your brain? Well, before we head off on a guided tour of the complex components within your brain, take a quick moment to try out this true-or-false quiz to see if you're really a whiz.

The *How Well Do I Know My Brain* Quiz

Mark these statements as true or false:

1. During the last 200,000 years, the human brain has evolved significantly. T/F
2. When we are born, the brain is already fully formed and not able to change much from there. T/F
3. There are 500 million neurons in the human brain. T/F
4. In the basal ganglia you will find at least 50 percent of the neurons present in your brain. T/F
5. The limbic system is the most recently evolved part of the brain. T/F
6. The cerebellum is known as the CEO of the brain. T/F

Answer Key

1. F: Since the human brain has not changed significantly during the past 200,000 years, you will find that the instinctual (or reactive) brain often takes precedence over your prefrontal cortex, which is your thinking (or rational) brain.
2. F: Although this was the common scientific belief for years, recently they have discovered that your brain is able to change—throughout your life.
3. F: Much more than 500 million. The average brain consists of more than 86 billion neurons, in addition to billions of "helper" cells.
4. F: It's the cerebellum, often referred to as your "little brain," that contains 50 percent of the neurons in your brain. There are 69 billion cerebellar neurons in the average brain.
5. F: The frontal lobe is the most recently evolved part of your brain. This is the part that really makes you human because it allows for conscious thought, planning, and impulse control.
6. F: An area of the frontal lobe, called the prefrontal cortex (PFC), is known as the CEO of your brain. The PFC integrates sensory information with decision-making and action-taking.

YOUR BRAIN PORTFOLIO

The most basic of all parts of the brain also happens to be the most crucial part of a healthy brain. That is the brain cell known as the neuron, along with its billions of helper cells, such as glia and astrocytes. The average brain is made up of more than 86 billion neurons with billions of additional helper cells with a primary function of forming synapses that are crucial for the exchange of electrical and chemical information.

Sounds like it could get messy up there, but those neurons are organized well, and don't just relay information at random. Your brain is arranged into different regions, each specializing in certain types of information—from information necessary for survival to information about your body's overall health status, all the way to more complex regions that are concerned with your deep thoughts and emotions.

The Synapse

Every neuron has a soma, or a central body, that contains the nucleus, or control center. Connected to the top of the soma, each neuron has a network of branches called dendrites that form a complex dendritic "tree." On the bottom of the soma, each neuron has a single, long projection called an axon that signals to other neurons. An electrical impulse, called an action potential, is propagated from the dendrites to the tip of the axon. The space between two neurons communicating—whether it be axon to dendrite, dendrite to dendrite, or axon to axon—is called the synapse. Chemical messengers called neurotransmitters can be released across the synapse and bind to the nearby axon or dendrite. These neurotransmitters help filter information, and increase the likelihood of the neuron relaying the action potential, and information, to another neuron, or inhibit it from "talking" to another neuron completely. Each neuron can make between 1,000 and 15,000 synapses, which, for all neuron in the brain combined, is an extensive network of approximately 100 trillion synapses.

The Three Sections of Your Brain

Generally speaking, there are three major sections within the brain, each with many structures working together for a common goal:

1. **Hindbrain.** This is the brain area responsible for controlling basic body functions that we don't need to think about to regulate but are crucial to our survival. These include functions like breathing, heart beat, sleep, balance, and swallowing. This area makes sure that all involuntary responses that result in normal body function work as they should, without you even knowing it.
2. **Midbrain**. This area sits just in front of your hindbrain and plays a role in motor control, vision, hearing, and regulation of body temperature and it also helps you go to and stay asleep. The midbrain also releases neurotransmitters responsible for motivation of basic motor responses like eating or drinking.
3. **Forebrain**. The forebrain is the largest area of the brain in humans, sitting on top of the midbrain and containing the cortex, limbic system, and relay centers. It is responsible for processing sensory information, like seeing and hearing; producing conscious thought; forming memories and feeling emotions; and initiating behaviors based on conscious decisions. The forebrain, because of the neocortex, is known as your "higher" brain. It's the part you have probably seen a million pictures of and it somewhat resembles a wrinkled looking mushroom cap (the wrinkles increase your brain's surface area, meaning that you can pack more neurons inside, which allows you to learn and make new connections). The neocortex has the responsibility of planning, along with creating abstract thoughts and reasoning. This is the part of your brain tasked with sensing the world around you and integrating the information from your different senses. It allows you to devise

reactions, and think about the act of thinking. This region is responsible for creating your personality, establishing hopes and dreams, and your ability to speak. The forebrain also contains the limbic system, which contains structures responsible for experiencing feelings like pleasure and aversion, or happiness and fear. The limbic system is highly responsive to hormones and drugs and can be easily manipulated by sensory inputs like sight or smell. This is the brain region that makes you want to buy food when you see a commercial for it. Not only does this brain region help you experience feelings, it motivates behaviors directed to make those feelings happen again if positive or to be avoided if negative.

YOUR FOREBRAIN: ITS FOUR AREAS AND WHAT THEY DO

The forebrain is a rather large area of the brain, containing many of your highest-order functions. To help classify and organize the cortex, neuroscientists have split the forebrain into four lobes: frontal, temporal, parietal, and occipital.

There is even further division within each of these lobes. They are separated into left and right halves, also known as hemispheres, by the central sulcus, the major groove running lengthwise along the center of your brain. While these hemispheres mostly share the same function, they are responsible for these functions on opposite sides of your body. Interestingly, for the most part, the right side of the brain handles the left side of the body, while the left side of the brain takes care of the right side of the body.

It's complicated, but hang in there and we'll describe the roles that each of these lobes play. Becoming familiar with the various parts of your brain will really increase your understanding of how the brain functions overall, as well as what can be done to protect and encourage your brain's functions to harness its power and get you thin.

Frontal Lobe

Sitting front and center in your brain is the area called the frontal lobe. Comprising around 30 percent of the total size of your brain, this is the largest and most evolved part of your brain; it's really the part of the brain that makes you human. It's responsible for most decision making, it gives the core of your personality, and it lets you think about yourself as a person. These are some pretty important roles, so you could even say that this lobe acts as the CEO, checking on all your decision making and providing the final okay to your actions—including those used for weight loss—before you make them.

Prefrontal Cortex

Within the frontal lobe, right at the forefront, is the prefrontal cortex (PFC), which is also split down the middle into left and right hemispheres. You will find the PFC just behind the middle of your forehead. This area is the last to develop when you became an adult. Teenagers certainly like to think they already have a fully developed brain, but in reality the prefrontal cortex hasn't finished growing yet, and won't reach its peak until after adolescence. There are slight gender differences with this process between the two genders. It will start and finish developing around a year earlier for girls.

Your prefrontal cortex operates as the hub for all brain-mind functions. Basically, this does more than just regulate signals transmitted by neurons to other areas of the brain and your body. It also allows you to have an awareness of what you are physically doing, and lets you reflect on these actions. The PFC allows for control of emotional responses, which is done with connections to your deep limbic brain, giving you the capability of focusing on anything you pick and allowing you to gain insight about your own thinking. The PFC is unique because it is the only part that has the power to control your emotions and behaviors and helps you focus on any goals you may pursue. It lets you take charge of what you want and how you go about getting it! The PFC has several subdivisions designated for taking on distinct types of decision making. The subdivisions include:

1. Your ventral medial PFC plays a major role in regulating your emotions and assessing risks, which means that this area plays a role in decision making for food habits in response to emotional stimuli. Depression and various similar mood states are associated with overeating, resulting in increased BMIs.
2. Your orbitofrontal cortex (OFC) is part of your PFC, and is defined anatomically as the area within the PFC sitting directly above the eye orbits—which, of course, is where it gets its name. Your OFC handles more of the evaluative tasks and looks to place an actual *value* on something. It's responsible for decision making in selecting which option out of a few is best for *you*! It also helps you conceive an adequate expectation for all consequences (both good and bad).
3. Your medial PFC works to keep both the OFC and ventral medial PFC under control by effectively serving up a dose of fear into other regions, which may be fired up. It can even put an end to your weight loss dreams . . . if you let it!

Since the PFC is, in essence, in control of your brain, the more you become familiar with all of the departments within your PFC, the more likely you will be to make wise and productive decisions—especially when it comes to food and exercise. The PFC can be an asset in making wise decisions because it acts as your emotional and logical arbitrator, rather than jumping to make decisions based on fear.

Temporal Lobe

The temporal lobe is situated under your temples on both sides of your head, and just behind (as well as below) the frontal cortex; this winds up making two separate temporal cortices. Your temporal lobes play a role in some sensory processing, for example hearing, and they're also the lobes involved with both speaking and understanding speech. In both of the temporal lobes you will find a brain structure known as the hippocampus, which is important for learning and memory as well as regulation of mood. The hippocampus is required for you to form new factual or emotional experiences. Your temporal lobe functions as the entryway to your thoughts and experiences and helps determine how they are processed for storage in your mind. Damage to this area results in problems storing memories.

Parietal Lobe

Next we have the parietal lobe. The two halves of this region sit at the top of your brain, in the area just behind the frontal lobe and above the temporal lobes. Here your brain integrates information received from the senses including vision, touch, balance, and hearing. Your parietal lobes also provide you with a sense of location—known to neuroscientists as *proprioception*—which is how you know where in the world you are located. Basically, this helps you move through your daily life without hitting any walls.

Occipital Lobe

Each of the two occipital lobes is found at the back of your head, sitting just behind and below the parietal lobes. This part of the brain handles the processing all of visual information that enters your brain from your eyes. Since we most often rely on our vision over any of the other senses, this entire lobe of the brain is specifically dedicated to processing all the visual information. This is especially important when it comes to weight loss as visual cues play a role in what we want to eat, what we like to eat, and even when we eat.

Cerebellum

The cerebellum, which is sometimes referred to as your "little brain," is located under the occipital lobes and parietal lobes and is really a distinct area separate from the four lobes. Amazingly, 50 percent of all neurons in the brain are contained in this tiny region. This portion of the brain plays a major role in motor control, as well as attention and language.

With the cerebellum, most of the input is focused on adjusting your actions to what's going on in the outside world and making sure you are coordinated in everyday movements, including body posture during walking, eye movements, and hand tracking. It handles the computation of a lot of information in a very tiny space. Recently, neuroscientists have begun to understand that the cerebellum is also crucial in other processes associated with learning, most of which occur subconsciously. For example, a professional basketball player dribbling the ball down the court uses his cerebellum in a similar way that you would when responding to an unexpected, loud noise by reflexively jumping. Both of these body responses stem from action patterns that depend on the cerebellum, just the same as many of your fundamental emotional responses.

Hippocampus

Short-term memories are made in your hippocampus. Some of those memories will be made into long-term memories if they are determined to be important enough. Memories of failed weight loss attempts and "dieting" gone wrong, where you have felt moody and lethargic, can fill your hippocampus and result in a mental standstill when it comes to starting on a new weight loss plan. Don't let an overactive hippocampus stop you from being successful. To retrain your brain, you can fill your hippocampus with positive memories associated with eating healthy, delicious meals and successful workouts that made you feel good about yourself. Over the next few chapters there will be many ideas provided for working with your stored memories.

DEEPER BRAIN STRUCTURES

Much attention tends to focus on the neocortex because it is a large component of the brain and it is responsible for the functions that you are most familiar with, like how you think about yourself and make connections to the world around you. It also manages speech, comprehension of complex concepts, and abstract thought.

Since it is responsible for so many of the things that you are aware of each and every day, you would think that the neocortex takes up the most space in the brain; in fact, it only makes up one-third of your brain. The other two-thirds of your brain—sometimes known as "deep" brain areas, hidden buried below the neocortex—hold the key to even more important functions such as learning and memory. Underneath the neocortex you will find most of your emotional brain areas, better known as the limbic system.

Anterior Cingulate Cortex

Your anterior cingulate cortex (ACC) contains neurons known as "spindle cells." These cells are unique within the animal world, and only humans, great apes, elephants, and a few whale species have them. Interestingly, humans have the most out of all these animals, with twice as many as great apes. Spindle cells are regarded as important for the evolution and higher function of the human brain. Spindle cells assist information as it travels from the back to the front of your brain. These cells are critical in helping your ACC focus attention, exert self-control, and spot errors from a range of sources all at the same time.

The anterior cingulate cortex is located between the decision-maker area of the frontal cortex and the emotional region, or limbic brain. Here it fills its role in emotional activities, taking information about emotions, empathy, and reward from the lower limbic brain structures over to the prefrontal cortex. After the prefrontal cortex processes the information, a reaction to the processed information, along with a plan of action, is delivered back through the anterior cingulate cortex to the limbic brain. Think of this part of your brain as the "problem solver," the middle man between your emotional self and your rational self.

You can train your brain by learning to how to strengthen your prefrontal cortex's skills in controlling your emotional responses (which you will learn more about in Chapters 4 and 5). When you do this successfully, you will increase the neuronal connections directed back down in an effort to suppress negative or undesirable emotional states coming from the deeper limbic structures. Accomplishing this allows your brain to better make goal-oriented, rather than emotionally driven, decisions.

Deep Limbic System

In a small area, about the size of a walnut, connected to the anterior cingulate cortex, you will find the thalamus, hypothalamus, and amygdala. Each has unique and important functions:

- **Thalamus:** This can be found at the top of the brain stem. It relays messages coming from the spinal cord, traveling up to the cerebrum, and then back down the spinal cord to your nervous system. The thalamus also regulates the activity of the cortex via the reticular activating system and can modulate feelings and emotions through this pathway.
- **Hypothalamus:** This area is also located at the base of the brain. It plays a big role in monitoring and maintaining many important functions in the human body, including those related to managing your weight. The four major functions of the hypothalamus are feeding, fighting, fleeing, and reproducing. The hypothalamus regulates hormones and controls appetite, thirst, sleep, body temperature, and circadian rhythms.

- **Amygdala:** Located deep at the center of your limbic brain, this region is no bigger than an almond. It controls many basic and emotionally charged needs. It generates strong emotions—including fear, anger, hate, lust, and love. Dysfunction of the amygdala has been linked to depression and addiction.

Your Amygdala and Food Responses

Although the amygdala is often associated with memory formation in regards to emotions, it also plays a role in the process of eating. The amygdala is tasked with perceiving taste within foods, which in turn results in our desire to eat more or less of a food. While there is still a lot to investigate on the role of the brain in food intake, studies have shown that stress does play a role in the response of the brain to food-related cues, and this results in an increased response in the amygdala, similar to what is seen among obese individuals. Since this is where pleasure sensations play a role, triggering the amygdala could have a negative impact on your trek to getting thin.

The deep limbic system is actually quite old in terms of that part of the mammalian brain, and was the first piece that allowed us to experience and show our emotions. It is responsible for all emotional associations, like being passionate about something or lusting after something, all of which spice up our lives whether they be positive or negative. Since this part of your brain is tied to emotional responses, including fear and pleasure, learning to quiet your amygdala will help you to make better decisions about behaviors associated with food choices, especially in relation to emotional triggers. (You will learn how to do this in Chapter 4.)

Generally, when your deep limbic system is silenced, or becomes less active, you can experience a positive state of mind because you can't feel negative emotions like fear, aggression, anxiety or hatred. However, the reverse is also possible. When your deep limbic system is pumped up, or overactive, negative emotions like anxiety and fear take the lead. Emotional regulation of sensory information from the amygdala is critical because it dictates the importance that you place on events in your life that thrust you into action (such as pursuing things that bring you happiness) or that cause you to avoid things (like pulling away from something that has brought you pain or disappointment in the past).

Basal Ganglia

Your basal ganglia are a series of brain areas, known as "nuclei," that are grouped into two sets, each with distinct functions:

The first set, which includes the striatum, pallidum, substantia nigra, and subthalamic nucleus, is involved with motor control. At this time, these basal ganglia regions are suspected to primarily play a role in "action selection," which basically means that they help you quickly decide which out of a few possible ways you should react in a situation. Your basal ganglia can promote your survival by guiding your movement away from, as opposed to closer to, a speeding car while you're cross the street.

The second set of nuclei, altogether referred to as the limbic nuclei of the basal ganglia, contains the nucleus accumbens, the ventral pallidum, and the ventral tegmental area (VTA). These sections play a vital role when it comes to determining the sensations of anxiety and reward, especially though the connections among the ventral tegmental area and the nucleus accumbens. Your nucleus accumbens, often referred to as your "pleasure center," is stimulated at times when you are either anticipating or actually experiencing something pleasurable or rewarding. More intense neuronal firing corresponds with increased desirable anticipation of the outcome. It also relates learned events against potential outcomes in the future. Overstimulation of this area may lead to unrestrained overindulgence or perhaps go as far as addiction. Activity of the ventral tegmental area also regulates reward because dopamine cells in the VTA synapse on neurons in the nucleus accumbens and excite them. Discipline and caution are the focal counterpoints to an overcharged reward center. Many addictive drugs, like cocaine and nicotine, affect this pathway, along with natural rewards like savoring a delicious meal. The more pleasurable the reward, the higher the activity of the circuitry between the VTA and the nucleus accumbens.

Food Addiction?

You may know a little about drugs and the addictive power they have, but who would have thought that some foods could trigger the same kind of response? Recent neuroscience research indicates that fatty foods set off the same pleasure-seeking regions of the brain that are commonly activated in drug addicts, leading to the new thought that food can be addictive. Just like with drug addictions, researchers found that pleasure centers in the brain lose their responsiveness over time, meaning that it takes more and more of the "substance" to feel fulfilled. While the initial research was completed using rats, the studies give promising new insight into ways we can address obesity, or any excess weight.

CHEMICAL MESSENGERS

Your brain contains a complex network of neurons. Their whole purpose is to transmit signals between the cells. These signals are transported electrically within a single neuron and then transported chemically between the neurons. So, what's responsible for delivering those chemical messages? Neurotransmitters, of which there are many different types. Some will transport fairly straightforward, basic messages; others are much more complex. These complex neurotransmitters have different functions spread all over different brain regions, and these are often termed *neuromodulators*. Do you recognize the terms dopamine, serotonin, and acetylcholine? They are three of the more commonly known neuromodulators. Acetylcholine has been shown to have an importance in shifting from the sleep state to an awake state, plus it aids in maintaining your attention and memory formation. Both dopamine and serotonin are known to be vital neurotransmitters when it comes to the regulation of mood, pleasure, happiness, and rewarding situations. In addition, serotonin is among the more important neurotransmitters when it comes to your body weight, because at normal levels it improves mood and prevents carbohydrate cravings. It seems that both dopamine and serotonin are natural appetite suppressants. Judith Wurtman, PhD, has researched the role of carbohydrates, serotonin, and weight management. Using earlier discoveries that serotonin can only be created after carbohydrates were consumed, this research monitored participants after they consumed a carbohydrate-containing drink before they ate their meal and found that those participants were better in control of their appetite and overall calorie intake. Conversely, those drinking a protein-containing drink did not demonstrate this same decrease in appetite. This just goes to show you the power of keeping those neurotransmitters, especially serotonin, in balance if you want to control your weight, and it seems that your diet may even play a role in keeping those serotonin levels in check.

Changing the number of these neurotransmitters can be helpful for getting what you want out of a situation. The best way to go about this would be to decrease those neuromodulators that bring about negative feelings and increase those that can impact you in a positive way. Exercise is one way that can help you increase those neurotransmitters that have a positive effect. It is also good to know that you don't even have to make a big change in the number of neuromodulators transmitting signals between neurons to have a visible outcome, either positive or negative, on your mood and temperament. Changes that alter the balance of serotonin and other neurotransmitters in your brain may lead to mood disorders such as depression, panic attacks, anxiety, and phobias. Therefore, it's essential to have the right balance of these neurotransmitters in order for your brain to buzz along, operating at an optimal level with *you* in the driver's seat.

Now that your brain is in full gear, let's head on over to the next chapter, where you'll get a lesson on the recent neuroscience breakthroughs that will help you to get thin!

CHAPTER 3

YOUR THIN QUEST DEPENDS ON RECENT BREAKTHROUGHS IN NEUROSCIENCE

Principle: Advancements in the field of neuroscience bring new knowledge, which may be the key to maximizing your brainpower and getting thin.

Neuroscientists have uncovered new insights into the human brain and its capabilities in just the last decade. In this chapter, you'll take a look at the insights and recent discoveries that will be the most relevant to you as you seek out your thin body, including information on how to rewire the circuitry of your brain and restrain oversensitive emotions, as well as use your imagination to help create your own reality. You may not realize it, but your brain is more able to adapt than you probably have thought. In fact, your mind (your thoughts) has the power to control your brain (the structural parts), turning it into your diligent weight loss partner, as you'll come to learn from your reading in this book.

Previously, scientists held the thought that the human brain and brain structures were formed early on—starting when you were a developing fetus in the womb and continuing throughout childhood. The thinking was that you only had so many neurons in each specific brain structure, and that as soon as you finished developing in childhood you were unable to make new connections. Basically, brain growth was believed to have ended at that time and didn't continue into adulthood. However, in the last decade, researchers have discovered significant new evidence that what they previously believed about this was, in fact, not true, and that something known as *neuroplasticity* continues over the whole course of our lives.

MOLD YOUR BRAIN

In neuroscience the word "plastic" is used to refer to a material that can change and has the possibility to be molded into something new. Neuroplasticity is the ability of your brain to change into something new, or change its shape. In fact, scientists have new knowledge indicating that throughout the course of your life, your brain can continue to:

1. **Start up dormant circuitry.** Most of the time something you have learned or a skill you developed doesn't get fully forgotten, but rather becomes dormant. With just a little practice, your neurons are kicked back into gear. It's just like riding a bike!
2. **Generate new circuitry.** When you're taught something new, your brain has the ability to strengthen neuronal connections that you already have and, from there, form new synapses—which allows you to get the most out of those new skills. You can also build neuronal circuitry to inhibit yourself from doing old, destructive behaviors.
3. **Rewire circuitry.** When your brain rewires its circuitry, it basically reassigns tasks. You can rewire one part of a neural pathway that has been used for one task to take on a different task. One example of this is with stroke patients who are able to relearn certain tasks, like how to feed themselves, despite having had some of their neurons destroyed.
4. **Quiet abnormal circuits.** Abnormal circuits are found in conditions like phobias, post-traumatic stress disorder (PTSD), obsessive-compulsive disorder (OCD), depression, and other

similar conditions. It is possible for some parts of your brain to wield control over other parts. In turn, this can alter how much of an affect they have on your mood and thought processes. Negative thought patterns and habits can be inhibited.

All of this means that, throughout your life, you can constantly train your brain to focus on weight loss! How does this work? Read on . . . .

How Can Neuroplasticity Help You Get Thin?

With neuroplasticity, you have the power to train your brain to do whatever it needs to do, no matter how old you are. Here's why:

1. **Your actions can impact the different regions of your brain by revving up or holding back circuits.** Example: If you get annoyed anytime someone brings donuts to work, you are activating certain brain pathways out of habit. However, you can learn how to retrain your brain to put an end to these pathways while you learn to strengthen others. That way you don't automatically jump right to the "annoyed" state the moment you find out that there's temptation down the hall. You can't make good food choices when your emotions are getting in the way.
2. **When you ask your brain to do more it will find available space to take on those new tasks by shrinking or repurposing space that has been tied up with tasks used less frequently.** Example: If you typically get depressed when you see your weight go up (even just a pound or two), your brain will hold on to that habit. If, however, you coach your brain to come up with new, positive reactions, like reminding yourself that weight can fluctuate daily and knowing you can make new choices the next day, you can put an end to those old pathways by making them less active, which opens up that space for new synapses and thought patterns. Your brain will now make creative connections so it can incorporate healthy changes into your daily routine.

3. **Your brain generally doesn't know the difference between your experiences and created fantasies.** Example: By filling your mind with pictures of you successfully reaching your goal weight, and visualizing these images long enough, your brain will interpret those images as if they really happened and you are already thin. Similarly, even thinking of doing bicep curls can activate muscle fibers.

Basically, your brain will strive to accomplish whatever you ask it to do. The more often you task your brain to dream up the thoughts that will help you get thin, the more your brain answers this call by generating new neuronal circuitry or ramping up what's already in place. This gets your brain working in positive ways to help you to become successful in weight loss, which in turn weakens those neuronal connections that empty your thin- and health-seeking notions.

Additionally, you are able to train your brain to flush away unproductive or defeating thoughts that pull you—and your brain—down, and instead light up your positive thoughts, which stimulates healthy thinking and makes you more productive and successful. You have the power to use your thoughts to lay the foundation for brain restructuring to get you to your thin self.

HAVE SUCCESSFUL THOUGHTS

Recent breakthroughs in neuroscience indicate something very exciting. Your thoughts are truly powerful. Just thinking them will help your brain to reshape itself, as well as create new synapses, which means that your thoughts are capable of helping you create new realities. Although outside factors can influence the thoughts that will reshape your brain, you don't need these outside factors to help you lose weight. Training your brain to work in a new way is easy if you think the right thoughts. You have the power to *will* your brain to do this. You just need to reinforce your new way of thinking—meaning your brain can change the way it functions to fall in sync with your desires and thoughts.

For example, scientific evidence tells us that if you picture what you want—often, and in detail—your dreams can become realities. So what does this mean for you? Basically everything that you think, do, or even say matters and impacts who you are from the outside in, all the way up to your brain. Therefore, just picturing your weight loss success or thinking about being successful at doing this will help you to achieve the reality of weight loss.

REVOLUTIONARY RESEARCH

New neuroscience studies are continuously demonstrating the inner workings of our brains. Let's spend a little bit of time looking at some of the revolutionary research that is helping experts better understand how you can train your brain to get thin.

The Impact of Valuation and Imagination on Decision Making

You can't make decisions without using the vital process of evaluation. No matter what decision you need to make—whether you're considering what to eat for dinner or determining your life goals—you need to include an evaluation of the situation. Research suggests that the brain's orbitofrontal cortex (OFC), a part of the PFC, plays an essential role in decision-making and expectations. The OFC seems to recognize "value" in a variety of forms, whether it's related to something directly impacting your survival (like food or water) or something more abstract (like poker chips). Most important, and really essential to this, is that recent research has confirmed that you can trigger the OFC, or any part for that matter, just by *imagining the value of something*. In a 2002 study completed by Dr. Nakia Gordon at Bowling Green State University, Ohio, it was reported that people have the ability to relive past events and experience emotions just by visualizing them along with the motions they performed while they were experiencing them. By the same token, a team headed by Dr. Will Cunningham from Ohio State University observed that when people think about things they place value in, the OFC becomes activated, which, in turn, means that you devote more of your neural circuitry and behavior to obtaining those things that you value. You can *assign* a value to anything you yearn for in life!

How Does the Evidence Weigh In?

Dr. Cunningham's study used young men as subjects, and asked them to picture things, people, or situations that they liked or disliked. They focused on the subjective value (quantity of their like or dislike) of each thing that they were imagining along with how much they really wanted it. Each area of the OFC lit up in response. This indicated to researchers that even though value doesn't always have a concrete number assigned, the OFC was able to take *any* valued idea set against *any* other valued idea and weigh them. This study also found an involvement of brain areas generally related to the generation of emotions along with OFC, despite participants being instructed to make decisions solely based on "value." Of course, since "value" is a subjective concept, it may involve sentimentality, fond memories, or even hate, which was taken into account for this imagination exercise.

In the Bowling Green study that looked at imagination and emotion, women who just imagined the act of laughing and crying showed activation in the same brain areas that would be activated in times when they were *really* laughing and crying. What does this mean? Simply *imagining* instances of joy or sorrow are indistinguishable within the brain from times when you are *really* experiencing these emotions.

Both the Bowling Green and Ohio State University studies demonstrate that simply *envisioning* valued things—people or experiences—free from external cues, will activate the brain in *exactly the same* way as really having those things or experiences. What does this mean for weight loss? Well, by visualizing your successful weight loss efforts you are more likely to find yourself reaching those weight loss goals. You see, you use the same regions in your brain while both actively working to lose weight and also while just visualizing those weight loss activities. You're Never Too Old to Learn Something New!

Neurogenesis, which literally means "birth of neurons," is the method by which new neurons form. While this phenomenon mostly occurs prior to birth, recent neuroscience research indicates that this process continues into adulthood, although in specialized regions. While this new idea of adult neurogenesis was slow to catch on, the shift in the neuroscience field has been taking hold. Let's take a look at the study results:

1. Going back to 1962, Dr. Joseph Altman, a neurobiologist, presented the first evidence of adult neurogenesis in the cerebral cortex of mammals. He provided solid evidence demonstrating how new neurons would form in the brain of adult rats subsequent to brain damage.
2. Then in 1963, Dr. Altman's initial study was followed up with similar displays of adult neurogenesis in the hippocampus, which is an area of the brain important for learning and memory.
3. Dr. Altman continued with his studies, and in 1969 he uncovered and named the source of adult-generated neurons in the olfactory bulb, which is responsible for your sense of smell. However, at the time, Dr. Altman's ground-breaking studies were by and large overlooked by the scientific community!
4. The good news is that in the late 1980s and the 1990s, Dr. Altman's research made a return to the spotlight when it was replicated and built upon by other neuroscience researchers, including Dr. Shirley Bayer, Dr. Michael Kaplan, and Dr.

> Fernando Nottebohm. Studying mammalian brains, as well as those of birds, these researchers demonstrated that adult neurogenesis does in fact occur in several areas of the brain in those animal species, and in the 1990s, adult neurogenesis in the human brain was confirmed.

These breakthrough studies shed new light on a great truth: *Your brain has the ability to generate new neurons.* Early studies may have demonstrated that this process happened in response to brain damage (like what is seen with a stroke), but additional studies demonstrate that new neurons can be generated in many animals as a result of new experiences and training routines. Even more exciting is that your neurons have the ability to *change.* Plasticity and a flexible nature allow neurons to strengthen connections within a short time (minutes). Can you believe it? In the short time it took you to read this paragraph, your brain can be on its way to a positive change, helping you become healthier and thinner!

Fire Together, Wire Together

In the well-known (to neuroscientists, that is) phrase by American neuroscientist Dr. Carla Shatz, "[N]eurons that fire together, wire together," we are reminded that neurons are essential to how we learn and how we make associations between various things. Canadian psychologist Dr. Donald Hebb developed what is now known as "Hebbian theory," that says that it is the *timing of when neurons fire that results in new or changed wiring.* Neurons that fire within rapid succession of each other, or just about the same time in response to a thought or encounter, will result in one of two possible outcomes. This will either strengthen preexisting synapses or create new synapses—which means that you can simply think about things and change your brain!

Dr. Hebb took what was known from many science disciplines and combined those data into a single statement: When neuron A is near neuron B, and neuron A is repeatedly stimulated enough to excite neuron B, some metabolic change occurs that makes neuron A more likely than any of the other neurons to stimulate neuron B. Basically, those two neurons end up more linked than the other neurons surrounding them, and the connection between those two neurons will be stronger than before that connection was made.

Focus on Getting Thin

Dr. Hebb's research has stood the test of time. After more than sixty years (his study was first published in 1949), and lots of experiments later, his theory remains fundamental to neuroscience. Based on what was discovered by Dr. Hebb and continued to be researched by other scientists, we see that continuous associations between neurons strengthen those associations. Let's look at an example: If you habitually focus on your past weight loss failures, unhappiness with your body, lack of self-confidence, and other negative thinking, the neurons responding to that specific mental activity will fire concurrently in a rapid nature, which will wind up automatically causing these neurons to start wiring together. Ultimately, this practice results in one more piece of neural structure that may cause you to feel like a failure, inadequate, or worthless.

Since that is the opposite of what you want to happen, you need to think about the positive. When you regularly zone in on those positive aspects of yourself and your body, the neurons included in *those* thoughts will be able to wire together, increasing connections, weaving together self-confidence, adequacy, and energy into the foundation of your brain, and stealing away synaptic strength from the negative paths.

Body Mindfulness

A prominent University of Wisconsin psychologist, Richard Davidson, PhD, has completed several studies looking at the effects of a practice known as mindfulness meditation, stemming from the

Buddhist technique of learning to center your mind by being fully present in the moment, or the here and now. Sounds interesting, right? Let's not get ahead of ourselves just yet. This meditation technique will be discussed in detail in Chapter 8, but first let's review Davidson's work and how this relates to the brain and getting thin.

In one of his studies, Davidson observed three distinct groups of people and their brain activity. This included a group of Tibetan Buddhist monks (who had spent countless hours practicing mindfulness meditation on compassion), people who had never meditated, and then people who took part in meditation training over a period of eight weeks. Davidson and his colleagues requested that the participants meditate, focusing on compassion and empathy, during which time he monitored their brains. Startling results revealed themselves to the researchers. Notably:

1. When subjects who had never meditated were asked to practice a traditional Buddhist compassion meditation, their limbic systems, which controls emotions, were stimulated during their first try.
2. When subjects who took part in the training began to meditate, their brains demonstrated more activity in the left prefrontal cortex (PFC). The PFC is not only the area of the brain thought to be responsible for producing positive emotions, but it's also an area that is very important in the decision making process. Interestingly, the left PFC as opposed to the right PFC is associated with more positive emotions. The left PFC can place a value on an emotional response, like happiness, resulting from getting a reward, like losing weight.
3. When the researchers reviewed the monks' brain scans, the results were shocking. The scans displayed significantly greater activity in their left PFCs, which could only be described as "well out of the normal range." Additionally, the monks demonstrated continued changes in their baseline brain func-

> tion indicating that their meditation practice influenced the way their brains functioned even when they were not actively meditating. Therefore, just by meditating, these monks *permanently* changed the level of activity in their PFC.

What can you learn from Davidson's studies? Even with little training, you can learn a technique that trains you to think differently, bulking up your neural connections in the area where it matters most: the CEO of the brain, the PFC. In just eight short weeks, people were able to rewire their brains as a result of training themselves to think in a new way.

The monks, who were well practiced in meditation, demonstrated even more differences in the brain. Unusually high activity in the monks' left PFC indicates that the monks formed new neuronal pathways as well as strengthened neural connections that already existed in this area in a unique manner—just by *thinking* about it. Their brains were wired for better decision-making capabilities and positive moods as a result of their meditation, for all hours of the day, even when not meditating. You have the ability to make this work for you, too! Mindfulness meditation could be the key to guiding you to make better decisions about your health, food choices, and level of physical activity, all by helping you to rewire, grow, and strengthen your PFC. So, what are you waiting for? Don't delay, your thin body is well within reach.

TIME TO GET TO WORK

By now you should have a basic understanding of the brain's regions along with its capabilities and shortfalls. Let's head off on the track to a new *thin* you by discussing the role your beliefs play in your brain's function, and how you can triumph over negative thoughts and reprogram your thinking patterns to shed those unwanted pounds.

CHAPTER 4

BELIEVE IN YOUR THIN SELF

Principle: Your brain believes those things you tell it to believe. If you believe in yourself, you are able train your brain to take a vital role in helping your *get thin* dreams become a reality.

Can you get thin? Of course you can! But this can't happen unless you—and your brain—truly believe it can happen. Your brain thinks, and it is heavily influenced by the messages you send to yourself and the actions that you take. It's possible that you have had negative thoughts about yourself and didn't even realize it. This chapter will help you learn about this hindering type of negative thinking (which really happens automatically) and the central beliefs you may have that could be leading you to these negative thought patterns. But don't worry! You'll also learn how to swap out those negative thoughts for positive thoughts—and associated actions—that will help you get your thoughts about your weight and weight loss on the track to success.

HOW DO YOU THINK ABOUT YOUR WEIGHT?

Recognizing your automatic thoughts about your weight, your body shape, and your weight loss goals can go a long way in helping you identify what you need to work on to be successful. Let's start by taking a quick assessment of how you think about weight.

The *How I Think about Weight* Quiz

1. I learned everything I know about weight and diet/nutrition:

A. by losing and gaining it over the years.

B. by listening to my friends and parents.

C. by reading books from credible sources.

2. When I think about a thin body shape, I:

A. just want it, and don't care how I get it.

B. want to look like my thin friends.

C. know where I am most comfortable and feel my best.

3. Thinking about losing weight makes me feel:

A. anxious and uncomfortable.

B. eager, but unsure of the next step.

C. energized and willing to work hard.

4. I believe that being thin is:

A. something that will make me feel good immediately.

B. something that comes naturally to some people, but not me.

C. something that requires hard work and dedication.

5. I think of myself as thin:

A. when I reach a certain number on the scale.

B. when my friends tell me I look good.

C. when I feel comfortable in my clothes and with how I look in the mirror.

6. I think being a healthy eater:

A. is hard work.

B. something that will come easier over time.

C. is easy with a little planning.

7. **When I see the number on the scale go down:**
   A. I reward myself with food.
   B. I reward myself with a treat, but not food.
   C. I pat myself on the back and feel good about my accomplishment.

Answer Key

If you chose mostly As, you have some dangerous thoughts when it comes to your awareness about weight and diet. You're letting your fears from past unsuccessful attempts hold you back and are likely letting instant gratification take over. This won't allow you to hold on to any weight loss success you have because you're less likely to make permanent changes. Your weight loss decisions are below your potential, but there's good news! You can significantly improve your diet and weight thoughts by reading this book and putting these tips into practice.

If you chose mostly Bs, your weight and diet awareness is on the outskirts. You have some solid knowledge but at times you seem to make your diet and lifestyle decisions based on emotional responses. As soon as you understand that you can toss out those emotional triggers and respond with a more logical reaction, you will find it easier to get what you want.

If you chose mostly Cs, you're in a prime position to make permanent changes now! You have a strong grip on the realities of weight loss and a healthy lifestyle, along with a healthy dose of motivation. You believe in hard work and know that it can pay off, but until now you've been cautious about taking action. With a little work fine-tuning your thoughts, you'll inspire yourself to turn your dreams into reality. You are ready to step up and take control of your weight.

THREE TYPES OF THOUGHTS

There are three basic thought patterns that your brain can use to decipher the world around you. These are automatic thoughts, assumptions, and core beliefs. In order to train your brain to get thin, you need to understand how these different thoughts initiate, how they impact whether you live your life in a positive or negative manner, how you select (consciously or unconsciously) the actions you take to lose weight, and how you can cultivate the type of control you need for your thoughts to train your brain to get thin. Let's take a closer look at each of these basic thought patterns.

Automatic Thoughts, on Autopilot

Automatic thoughts are those thoughts—whether conscious or unconscious—that you regard as true. When you have these thoughts, you're basically on autopilot when it comes to reacting to situations and events, which doesn't allow you to react with thoughtful analysis. Perhaps some of these sound familiar?

- I don't look good in this outfit.
- I can't trust my friend's opinions.
- I'm not creative.
- I'm not successful.
- I'm not really good at anything.
- I just can't learn how to eat the right foods.
- I find "diet" foods bland.
- I don't have any luck keeping the weight off.

While these thoughts may simplify your life by cutting back on some of the things you need to think about, they may also be working against you if they are self-limiting and simply not true.

Are You Functioning on Automatic Responses?

If you rely on these automatic responses to make it through your day, you may in fact be *healthy living* unconscious. You're *healthy living* unconscious if you:

- Resist facing your real health and weight status.
- Utilize defensive tactics, like denial.
- Let your unexamined views effect your food and exercise choices.
- Don't know what you should do in order to make healthy lifestyle decisions.
- Aren't employing all of your brain resources to help make realistic healthy decisions.
- Make emotionally based decisions.
- Aren't able to learn from past mistakes.

Being able to recognize when you're operating on autopilot gives you the power to stand up and take action, engaging your brain's CEO in the important task of healthy decision-making.

Automatic thoughts, whether conscious or unconscious, can increase your stress levels, which in turn causes your brain to release stress-related hormones such as cortisol. Cortisol has many negative effects on the body, which are detrimental to weight loss, such as increased storage of belly fat. An increase in cortisol produces a calamity of hormonal and neuronal changes that can hinder your judgment of many things, including making healthy lifestyle decisions. Fortunately, you have the ability to train your brain to curb those negative automatic thoughts and rewire itself for more positive forms of self-assurance that help focus your thoughts in a positive, supportive direction.

Assumptions

Thoughts that you have that developed from experiences or from beliefs that have been imposed on you or that others have influenced are known as assumptions. Just like with automatic thoughts, assumptions also act as a way for your brain to cut corners when interpreting what is currently occurring in your life or processing what may happen down the road. Assumptions, just like automatic thoughts, can be either conscious or unconscious. These assumptions are either created by you from past observations and experiences or based on what you have been taught by others as true. This means that the incorporation of your automatic thoughts in cooperation with your core beliefs will be the basis of what your brain deciphers as reality.

Have You Made These Assumptions?

- I made really healthy food choices all day so it doesn't matter what I eat for dinner.
- Since I have been eating the right foods, I can skip going to the gym for a few days.
- I would love to wear one size smaller jeans, but my body type won't let me.
- I'll never be able to get to that weight, so why should I work so hard?

Stand Up to Your Negative Assumptions

No one wants to have unnecessary worrying, fearful feelings even when you are safe, or holding back expressing your personality, but that's just what negative assumptions will do. Getting into the habit of always thinking the worst will happen can basically freeze up your brain when trying to determine positive solutions to get you to take positive actions.

Standing up to those assumptions that may be pushing you down a negative path will prep your brain for the new generation of neuronal pathways. The practice of meditation (as discussed in Chapter 8) can help you fight back those negative thoughts, swapping them out with positive thoughts by helping you live right here in the present. That is the right place to be to allow you to consciously decide how you think about what's going on at that moment rather than dragging up your past to get you to those unworkable conclusions. The creation and use of positive affirmations helps train your brain to visualize things in a much more positive manner.

Core Beliefs

Broad generalizations about how the world works, as well as about yourself, that your brain accepts as true, are known as core beliefs. These are what you rely on to interpret what happens in your life. Here are some examples of core beliefs with the potential to negatively affect your ability to get thin:

- I'm big boned so I will always be overweight.
- I don't have the ability to be successful.
- My metabolism is too slow to lose weight.
- I don't have any medical problems now so the excess weight isn't a problem.

No matter how illogical the underlying theories that form your core beliefs, they will effectively control your thought processes by strengthening what you already hold to be true. The end result is that your brain keeps heading down the same neuronal pathways that it has taken in the past, which creates even more of those synapses supporting your current, unhealthy core beliefs.

Core beliefs result in your brain responding with your same old go-to thought patterns when placed in new situations or experiences. Usually this happens so fast that you don't even question your reaction or response, and until something forces you to question those core beliefs, such as when something happens in your life that challenges those beliefs. This life occurrence doesn't need to be a negative one, either. A positive experience, such as achieving small weight loss by only making small changes, challenges your negative core beliefs and sends your brain reeling. Hopefully, you'll recognize that feeling as a positive thing and start to challenge those negative assumptions (in this example, the core belief that you have to do something drastic to lose weight) and trade those negative core beliefs for new, positive core beliefs.

The downside here is that your core beliefs are more deeply rooted in your brain than your automatic thoughts and assumptions, so they are much harder to change. But by working on your automatic thoughts and your assumptions you can reshape your core beliefs over time so that they become more positive and realistic. You have the power to chip away at those negative core beliefs and replace them with positive core beliefs, ultimately taking charge of your weight, changing your brain, and positively impacting your life.

THINK IT TO BE IT

Your thoughts shape who you are and what you do, in all aspects of your life. Every one of the actions you take is a consequence of your thoughts—so you need to *think it to be it*. Basically, what you think deep in your thoughts will be echoed in your life circumstances, and this happens because the changes you initiate in your life are always started by the changes you make in your thinking and how you perceive something.

Power Up with Positive Thoughts

Brain chemicals are released with every thought you have, so focusing on negative thoughts does a wonderful job of draining your brain's positive momentum. On the other hand, when you think positive and happy thoughts you decrease cortisol (the hormone released in response to stress) and increase the production of serotonin, which promotes your sense of well-being and happiness. This gets your brain functioning at its peak levels, which is definitely where you want to be when working on losing weight.

Why Optimism Pays

Optimists come out on top by thinking positive thoughts and believing in themselves. Optimists tend to be more confident and place trust in their capabilities, while pessimists tend to doubt what they are capable of accomplishing. What's more, scientists have found important differences between the optimists and pessimists.

Optimists credit positive events to themselves, listing their traits and skills as the reason that these positive events turned out that way. However, they label bad or negative events as temporary, often using words that indicate this is an occurrence just for the time being ("sometimes" or "lately"). The way they view life supports their quest for success by allowing them to:

- Better cope with the ups and downs we see in everyday life.
- View setbacks as something that they can conquer and attribute them to something external, not internal.
- Lead happy and fulfilling lives because they believe that they will lead happy and fulfilling lives.
- Develop healthy relationships with others, which help them in a variety of settings.
- Take better care of their physical and mental health.
- Live longer than pessimists.

Quite the opposite of optimists, pessimists believe good things that happen to them are not a result of something internal, but rather a fluke or occurrence brought on by an external influence.

They tend to see bad or negative events as a permanent state of being. Additionally, they:

- Automatically believe any setbacks they experience are permanent and result from their own failures.
- Experience higher rates of depression compared to optimists—they're about eight times more likely to be depressed.
- Have more relationship problems, which make it difficult to stay on track with healthy behaviors, since that requires a level of stability.

However, there is good news. You are in control and your mind is powerful enough to learn how to hold down those negative, pessimistic thoughts, while simultaneously pumping up your positive, optimistic thoughts. Even if you come from a pessimistic family, you still have the ability to change how your brain functions by creating neuronal blockades and reducing the neuronal patterns associated with negative thinking. While you may not have the power to completely override a genetic predisposition toward pessimism, you are able to drastically reduce its impact on your life.

THE INFLUENCE OF YOUR MOOD

Moods affect how your brain—and, really, your entire thought process—works. Having a positive mood leads to a more open mind so you are better able to react in a positive way. The same can be said for having a negative mood. When you are feeling down, your brain closes out your voice of reason and you are unable to take action or may react in a negative manner.

Surprisingly, negative moods do have a place in your life. These moods (or emotions) help you realize when you and your needs/values are not aligned. You should recognize those negative feelings as a way of alerting you that something may not be right and as a way to more completely recognize how you're truly feeling in a situation. It is really important that you are able to differentiate between those negative feelings that lead to changing your behavior in a positive way and those feelings that only undermine your ability to reach your true potential, and ultimately attain your goals. The better handle you have on those fearful situations, the better able you will be to suppress those feelings of fear and silence the amygdala, the part of your brain that associates fear with learning and memory.

PRACTICES GEARED AT CHANGING NEGATIVE THOUGHTS

If your life is run by negative thoughts, or if you're one of those people who always expects the worst outcome in any situation, then it's important for you to start anew, regroup, and take control of your thoughts. The good news is that you are able to rid yourself of those negative thought patterns by learning and applying a few easy practices. Let's discuss a few of these, like challenging absolutes, neutralizing negative self-talk, distracting your thoughts, and creating positive affirmations.

Practicing these techniques repeatedly will, over time, allow you to retrain your brain to work for you in a productive and positive way, leading you to expect the best outcomes in just about all situations. By being in control, you are the only one able to lead your brain to new ways to perceive situations and establish your expectations. Time to switch off your "autopilot" button and involve your brain in your quest to get thin.

Practice #1: Challenge Absolutes

You may have noticed that everyone has a tendency to think in absolutes: *If I don't fit into these pants, I won't go to the party.* Or, *If I don't eat as healthy as I planned this afternoon, I should just give up until tomorrow.* Well, thoughts like this may give you a laugh after the fact, once the panic subsides and you realize how silly they sounded—but when they happen, these are the kind of single-sided thoughts that result in unproductive habits. It is important to work on breaking these patterns. The next time you find yourself in a situation like this, take a moment to think about the thought and challenge those absolutes that your mind is busy generating. Then you'll want to jot down these thoughts to show yourself just how narrow your mind has become by writing the future before it happens. More often than not, you've blown the situation and resulting consequences way out of proportion. Each time you notice that you are thinking in these all-or-nothing terms, take a time-out to make a list of a variety of possible outcomes. This technique will help your brain create new and more creative solutions to these problems.

Practice # 2: Neutralize Negative Self-Talk

Almost everyone has his or her own version of negative self-talk: *Everyone has more willpower than I do. I just can't resist tempting foods. My genes won't let me lose weight.* If you happen to be one of those people, the time to pinpoint them and stand up to those internal, pesky voices is now. You will find that these thoughts tend to surface when you are experiencing feelings of insecurity, like when you are learning or trying something new. You might "hear" those inner voices chattering away with things like:

- "I'm not able to resist sweets when they are around."
- "I'm not good at cutting back on portions."
- "I'm never going to look good in those pants."

Challenge these thoughts head on and turn them around by declaring more realistic and positive thoughts:

- "I've passed by sweets before."
- "Last Thanksgiving, I didn't go back for seconds on the mashed potatoes."
- "I look really good in my favorite pair of black pants."

Repeating these positive thoughts frequently will cause your inner voice to support you and your quest for positive outcomes.

Practice #3: Distract Your Thoughts

Perhaps you are someone whose brain is packed with so many thoughts that you can't seem to focus. In that case, distracting your mind could be the trick you need to help put an end to all of that mindless obsessing over things you really have no control over or can't change.

It's easy to change: Get up and *do* something—anything—else that requires your undivided attention. Maybe you have a project you want to work on or maybe it's time to clean out your closet. Maybe it's dinnertime and you can focus on cooking a healthy meal or you have some spare time so you can fit in a workout. Whatever you can devote all of your concentration to is something that will positively distract your mind.

Practice #4: Creating Positive Affirmations

Don't let your negative thoughts take over your life! Instead, make a list of positive thoughts to oppose them. These positive affirmations should be specific and unique to each situation. Make sure they are detailed so your brain is better able to visualize these as already true. Replace your usual negative thinking in a situation with positive affirmations like:

- "It was really easy to work out at the gym today for an hour."
- "Having fruit after dinner for dessert really left me feeling satisfied."
- "It was a lot easier than I thought to pass on my morning donut."

Creating positive affirmations will help you relax your brain, which puts it in a healthier place to help you stick to your lifestyle modifications and operate at your maximum potential.

Saying these affirmations over and over throughout the course of the day will generate a mental picture of success so that your brain will be glad to satisfy your weight loss desires. At the very least, coming up with these positive affirmations will help to pacify your nerves, keeping you on track for better outcomes. Go ahead and test out those positive affirmations for the various situations that you find yourself in. Then sit back to take notice of how well your brain operates when you've given it orders to craft the perfect ending.

Once you have these positive affirmations created, write them on a piece of paper and take them with you everywhere you go. Then when a negative thought pops into your mind you are armed and dangerous. Simply review your affirmations and change the way your brain thinks and reacts in those situations.

MAKE POSITIVE ACTIONS OUT OF NEGATIVE THOUGHTS

One very effective way to train your brain is to allow yourself to take positive action. This way it will reinforce the kind of thought patterns you want to attain for healthy behaviors. Here are six trouble-free steps that you can take to make positive actions out of your negative thoughts:

1. Pinpoint both conscious and unconscious thoughts you may have, looking especially closely at those negative thoughts that are keeping your mind going round and round and never getting you where you need to be.
2. Neutralize negative thoughts by finding supporting evidence to contradict them.
3. Wrestle with the part of you that has confidence in those negative thoughts.
4. Find another explanation that disproves your original negative thought.

5. Don't be so judgmental—not just of yourself, but also of others.
6. Give validation to your positive thoughts and design scenarios where it's possible for you to re-experience them when needed.

In essence, you want to aim for the following:

- Find out exactly why you feel upset and/or think and behave in ways that are counterproductive for your goals.
- Get some insight into why it is that you think this way and address any underlying views you have about yourself and those around you, which may be keeping you down.
- Change your negative thought patterns and unrealistic views you may have that propel them.
- Learn to be objective when evaluating problems and circumstances.

Now take your current weight and lifestyle status, develop a list of positive points to counter those negative ones, and focus hard to purposefully see things in a more positive light. By doing this you will help train your brain to employ positive thinking more often.

TURN POSITIVE THOUGHTS INTO POSITIVE ACTIONS

By now you should have a good understanding of how you can train your brain in the art of thinking positive thoughts, so it's time to step it up and move on to the next level. Positive thoughts are the first step, but now you need to morph those positive thoughts into positive actions. As you start to take positive action in more and more situations, your brain will start to pool its resources and support you in morphing your ideas into reality to help you be successful, lose the weight, and get healthy. Don't forget that your brain is here to serve you, but it is you alone who can employ your mind to train your brain to get thin. Let's go over some methods you can utilize regularly to help take those positive actions.

Take Control of Your Subconscious

Don't discredit the power you have to control what your subconscious mind knows. Information flows in through your senses, but that doesn't mean that you can't allow your conscious mind to tell your subconscious mind how that information should be processed. You need to intentionally select a positive perspective in all situations you encounter.

Place Your Focus on Desired Outcomes

Make the most of your concentration skills and focus on your goals daily. Write out a list of actions you need to take to successfully achieve your goal. Read this before going to sleep each night, and then again each morning when you wake up. Sticky notes are perfect for putting these messages easily within view, whether you put them up on the bathroom mirror, your refrigerator, or your office workspace. Doing this will engage your mind to help you transform these into reality by fixing your mind on attaining your desired outcome. Repeating thoughts regularly will nestle them into your subconscious, and over time your subconscious will acknowledge and act upon them just the same as if they were true.

Mentally Picture the Desired Outcome

Mental pictures can (positively) deceive your subconscious into thinking your goal has already been reached, such as visualizing yourself fitting into your favorite bathing suit or favorite pair of jeans. Visualizations linked to emotion pull more weight, especially when they're linked to emotions that are positive. Once you have convinced your subconscious that your dream will come true and you're able to stick with those thoughts, your subconscious mind will turn your beliefs into actions. Have faith in your mind because it has the power to turn dreams into realities.

Obtain Specialized Knowledge

To be successful with weight management you need to learn as much as possible about healthy living, including diet (meaning what you eat or drink, not restricting foods to drop weight quickly) and exercise. The more time you can invest in seeking out credible sources and learning about health, eating properly, and exercising in a way that is appropriate for you, the more your brain will do as you wish by firing those existing synapses and then producing new synapses related to the gathering and processing of that knowledge. Ensuring that the learning process is pleasurable will aid in wiring positive feelings to positive action. Instead of dreading study time, remind yourself that this practice is inching you closer and closer to your goal. If you let this get you excited, your brain will take action appropriately—and positively!

MAKE IT A REALITY

Now that you've discovered ways to morph your thoughts into action, it's time to take the next step. You need to take your newly formed positive thoughts and apply them to create a more complete action plan—one that sends the loud and clear message that your brain needs to jump into action. Here's how you can do this:

- Pinpoint the strongest of your desires.
- Obsession! Once you are obsessed with achieving it, stay that way.
- Be specific about what you want and get this lined up in your sights.
- Be persistent in chasing your goal(s).

- Don't get stopped by obstacles. Find creative ways to conquer them.
- Persevere! Do not give in or give up.

You want to form neural pathways, so you need to really make conscious attempts at repeatedly reinforcing your goals. This will allow your brain to form, and start to prefer, the new neuronal pathway instead of habitually jumping into past, nonproductive responses. It takes at least three weeks to form a new, healthy habit.

CULTIVATE YOUR THOUGHTS

In order to have your thoughts flourish, much like fertile land, they must be cultivated. When you plant a seed, you want it to grow. A thought planted in your mind will only grow and strengthen if the proper care is given to help it sprout forth. Your thoughts can help you reach your dreams, or conversely can lead you to surrender to your fears. To achieve your healthy weight and best-looking body, you'll need to cultivate your mind's fertile land, weed out inhibiting thoughts, plant those hearty seeds, and then be prepared when the time comes to enjoy the fruits of your labor.

Now that you've taken the time to cultivate your land it's time to learn more about how to help these thoughts bloom. In the next chapter you'll see what you need to do to create your intention to get thin.

CHAPTER 5

CREATE THE INTENTION TO GET THIN

Principle: Defining your intentions will help your brain focus, sustain, monitor, and reward the completion of your goals that support your quest for weight loss success.

The key to achieving success when it comes to reaching your weight goals is having a clear definition of your intentions, the underlying reasons for why you want an outcome. In this case, your desired outcome is losing and maintaining a healthy weight. Knowing what you want to achieve and why is just as important as the road you will take to get there. In fact, you can't even start your journey without a deeper understanding of your intentions. These may be different for everyone, so don't be quick to judge others as you learn about their intentions. Simply focus on your own and know that if you have good reasons to want to get to that goal, you can focus your mind, and success will be yours.

To head off on your journey toward a healthy weight and that much-desired slender figure, the major questions you want to ask yourself are:

- Why do I want to lose weight?
- What will being thinner mean to me?

The answer to these two questions will help you begin the process of creating intentions. How? Because creating intentions specific to your individual quest for weight loss will result in your brain heading down the right path toward success. Don't let the intentions of others hinder your plans for getting thin. It is all too easy to become clouded by other people's reasons for your own weight loss. Remember, this is *your* journey. While friends and family are there for support along the way, cheering you on as you pass each milestone and shed each pound, you need to set the path in your brain based on your intentions.

TRUE INTENTIONS

As discussed in previous chapters, if you picture something hard enough, your brain will interpret this as truth, as though it had already happened. Keeping this in mind, you can see that the creation and the continual reinforcement of intentions is a powerful tool for setting up those neural pathways that you need to reach a healthy weight. This is why it is so important that you create those intentions with your own desires in mind. Working toward someone else's goals for you can backfire. Your intentions should be pure and clear and should set the tone for your own desires. This, in turn, will allow your brain to better focus on what you really want. The following quiz will help you begin the process.

The *Do I Know My True Intentions?* Quiz

1. I really want to lose weight because:

A. I want to live a longer, healthier life.
B. I want to fit in my favorite jeans again.
C. I want to have more energy to play with my kids or pets.
D. I want people to take me seriously.

2. When it comes to setting weight loss goals, I:

A. set long-term goals, perhaps with some short-term goals along the way.
B. focus on the numbers.
C. include my family as part of the process.
D. keep everything organized and charted, updating as necessary.

3. **The best thing that having weight loss goals does for me is:**
   - **A.** keep me in positive spirits.
   - **B.** help me visualize the outcomes and keep me focused.
   - **C.** help me keep my priorities.
   - **D.** offer a system of checks and balances.

4. **A typical weight loss goal for me would be:**
   - **A.** seeing a change in my Body Mass Index.
   - **B.** dropping one dress size.
   - **C.** losing five pounds this month so it's easier to stay active.
   - **D.** have my weight loss noticeable to others.

5. **When I accomplish a goal, I:**
   - **A.** celebrate my accomplishment by treating myself to something fun.
   - **B.** buy myself something nice.
   - **C.** celebrate with my family.
   - **D.** pat myself on the back.

Answer Key

If you chose mostly As, you have a good idea of the link between weight and health. You know that you want to live a long, healthy life, and that having a healthy weight is key to achieving those outcomes. You need think about how weight impacts how you feel and what goals you need to focus on to get yourself to a healthier place.

If you chose mostly Bs, you feel a strong connection between looking good on the outside and feeling good on the inside. While health may not be your first concern, you know that, in the long run, being healthier means that you can age gracefully. Just be careful—when you focus too hard on the visual outcomes, you can easily forget about your inner health, which is just as important.

If you chose mostly Cs, you are focused on your family and, while that is a good thing, you must really stop to think about how your family is influencing you. It is great to want to lose weight so that you can be better able to spend quality time with your family, but you need to make sure that your desires, not pressure from your family, inspire you to lose unhealthy weight.

If you chose mostly Ds, you tend to be more of a people pleaser. When it comes to weight loss you want to look good and put your best foot forward, especially when it comes to being taken seriously in the professional world. Making others happy with the things you do in turn makes you feel proud of your accomplishments, and can work in a positive way to keep you in track. To achieve your greatest success, think about who you are really trying to please and why.

IDENTIFY YOUR INSPIRATION

Henry Ford once said, "There is no happiness except in the realization that we have accomplished something." The things that inspire you will propel you toward your weight loss goal, and this accomplishment will bring you happiness that will run over into other aspects of your life. Keep in mind that success happens when you are invested in an outcome and that, to be successful, something needs to excite you. You can't just pick something random to focus on and be successful with it. It needs to have meaning. Success comes from things into which you have invested time and energy, where you have given deep thought to what matters. Things you care about will result in success over time. For success in weight loss, you need to figure out what excites you, or rather what is inspiring you to lose the weight. There will definitely be something that is sparking your interest in dropping those pounds. You just need to identify these inspirations within yourself and find meaning in these in order to be truly successful on your journey to get thin.

Once you determine the whys in your weight loss goals—*Why do I want to lose weight? Why do I want to wear those jeans? Why do I want to change my diet and lifestyle?*—then determining your true intentions for weight loss will come easily. Your answers to these questions will guide you there. Your inspiration is essential to sticking with your goals. Not only do these inspirations fuel what you do with your body, but they are also the focus of your mind. Inspiration for weight loss means there is something pushing you in a positive way to be the best you can be. This powers your mind to get the message that something is meaningful to you. The inspiration you have for your weight loss will make sure you have clearly defined intentions for your quest to be thin, and in the end will help you to achieve the best outcomes.

Create Your Get Thin Mission Statement

Let's start with setting a mission statement. This is similar to a mission statement you might find for a business, but in this case, it is all about you. Aim for something realistic, but that still captures who you are, your values in life, and what you're setting out to achieve. This is more than just a message stating your goals. Think bigger! This is your intention for losing weight and it will serve as a motivator as you shed pounds and stay on course for your weight loss goals. Once you have reviewed and refined your intentions, write them on a 4"× 6" index card and tape this to a location that you see daily, like a bathroom mirror or closet door.

Defining your intention will naturally guide you to setting goals to get you on your way. It's hard to set short-term weight loss goals if you really have no idea what is triggering you to want to lose weight. But if you know that, then you are headed in the right direction. These are the first steps on your path to losing weight, and looking and feeling your best. So defining and putting your intentions down in a mission statement is the first step toward weight loss because mission statements:

- Allow your brain to focus on the actual act of losing the weight.
- Narrow your field of awareness, which helps your brain direct its energy toward shedding the extra pounds.
- Increase your perception of what's going on in your mind.
- Help you stay in the present, focused on what needs to happen at this very moment to help you lose weight.
- Help you reflect on what works and what doesn't work.
- Let you see and address any possible resistance to losing weight.

Keep in mind that people change over time, so this means that your intentions will change too. But for right this moment, knowing your intentions will help your brain to focus its resources to help you discover and maximize pathways to success. Now that you know how your intentions affect your mind, let's move on and discuss their specific role on your brain.

PAY ATTENTION TO YOUR BODY

Your brain's reticular formation directs incoming stimuli to your conscious or unconscious mind, acting like a gatekeeper. This in turn allows you to tune in to whatever you decide is important. At the same time, it is able to tune out what you deem to be unimportant. It may seem complex, but having an understanding of this process will ensure that you are paying attention to the things that will help lose weight.

To fire up your reticular formation in an effort to make sure information (stimuli) gets processed correctly, focus on what you want. This means establishing what it is you really and truly desire. Now is the time to get really specific. This means knowing exactly what you want and why. You are in control. By narrowing your focus, you will engage your reticular formation and help block out any distractions. Keeping out thoughts that aren't part of what you find to be important and in need of your attention will ensure that you are correctly focused on what it is you truly want and desire.

What Motivates You?

Desiring a thin physique isn't solely about the number on the scale. It's about health, pride, self-control, being energetic, feeling good, and having confidence, to name a few motivational targets. The emotions you have about being thin can be extremely complex. These are shaped and impacted by family history of weight, cultural perceptions of weight, personal beliefs on weight loss, food preferences, and geographic region. To help your brain work hard toward losing weight and getting thin, identify and focus on what motivates you. Think about what sets your passion on fire and pushes you toward your goals. Doing so helps your brain conjure up those motivations when it's time to focus on important decisions like what you should eat for lunch or passing up the donuts someone brought into work that morning.

Unite Your Best Body Consciousness

It shouldn't be surprising that, if your consciousness is divided, it's nearly impossible for your mind to best interpret your desires. An intention that isn't steadfast won't motivate your subconscious to give you the energy you'll need to really turn that intention into reality. One essential aspect of learning to harness your consciousness to achieve your dreams is making sure that your thoughts are consistent. When you have consistency in your thoughts, your goal will be better received. On the other hand, when you have inconsistencies in your thoughts about what you want in life, often flip-flopping on your dreams or desires, your energy will be wasted. This will then result in a defeated feeling; you may feel frustrated and maybe even a little annoyed. Train your brain to work *with* you, not against you, by shaping your intentions. You want to be clear and consistent, keeping your brain focused on what you really want. Creating goals is the best way to find what actions and steps you need to take to move you closer to your intention of getting thin, and staying that way.

UNDERSTAND YOUR VALUES

Your brain needs specifics, so in addition to defining your intentions, you will want to take some time to identify your core values —the basis of your intentions that will ultimately set you up for long-term success and a lifetime of happiness. A value is defined as something that you appreciate, something you consider desirable, or something that you have placed some sort of worth or price on (although not necessarily financial). Your core values are the values that provide you with the foundation for all that you do, right down to the reasons why you want to lose weight. These values help to guide us in the decision-making process and prevent us from doing things that go against what we truly believe in. This is why our intentions are so important. Knowing what we want and how to get it is dependent upon what we value or hold dear to us. Working toward a weight loss goal, a great-looking body, and feeling good about yourself inside and out, will all hinge on how your values—the next step on your path to creating achievable goals—play a role in what you wish to achieve.

Values Differ

Reasons for losing weight will be different for everyone and the things that you specifically hold in high regard or place a value on will determine how you go about your weight loss. Whether you're losing weight for your health, family, or a successful career, your main values will play a central role in setting your goals. Even values like honesty, trust, hard work, and determination will factor in to how you go about setting your goals. Other core values may include autonomy, excitement, and spirituality. There really are many different values you may find that are important to you, so it is important to know what it is that you truly value in your life. These values are yours and yours alone, and it's only natural that they will be different for everyone. Don't make the mistake of letting the things that someone else values determine how you go about setting your weight loss goals.

The most successful people are those who have a good understanding of themselves and their values. It's one reason they are able to set realistic goals and find themselves making it all the way to the finish line. You can get there, too; you just need to get off on the right foot, and this starts by knowing what values you need and want to live by.

Identify Your Values

Quickly, without overthinking, jot down a list of your core values. Again, these values can be anything from family to independence to honesty. Write down as many can come up with. Keep polishing and reworking these until you have a concrete list of at least five core values that you know deep in your heart play an essential role in how you live your life.

Once you have your weight loss mission statement (shaped by those intentions created earlier) and your five core values, it's time to set realistic, solid, and achievable goals.

CREATE GOALS

Those who never set goals risk living their lives without knowing what could have been. If you live this way, you'll only end up with a bunch of unanswered what-ifs. You can never be successful without setting clear goals because you won't have a clear way of measuring your success. That being said, setting goals for weight loss is not easy, and you can just as easily set up goals that just can't be achieved. Perhaps this is one reason why you have not met those weight loss goals in the past or have been unable to keep up with all the hard work you put in to getting those pounds off in the first place. It's easy to fall into this trap. However, now it's time to use your brain—and your body—to shed the weight once and for all.

Be Specific and Sincere

Knowing what you want is a key factor in being successful with weight loss. Your goals need to be specific and you must be honest with yourself in the goal-setting process. It is entirely possible that setting lofty goals, while they sound amazing, may not be realistic—you may be setting yourself up for failure. Since we all live in the real world, keeping goals realistic will help you better achieve success. Those intentions, based on your core values and grounded in sincerity with both yourself and your own capabilities will bring you that much closer to long-term success.

Goals may be the endpoint, but the process of getting there is important. This marks the roadmap you will follow all the way to the end. Goals act as something visible, something you can put in your sights, just off into the distance. Successful, long-term goals are the realization of your ideal body weight; short-term goals provide the key points along the path to get there. For example, a long-term goal may be to lose 40 pounds in the next year. To get here you will need some short-term goals to work at along the way. For this long-term goal, one short-term goal could be to get at least 150 minutes of exercise weekly. Knowing what you want and how to get it sends a clear message about what you want to achieve to your brain, firing up the neurons related to the task. There are certain steps you can take to create the goals that will greatly improve your chances of success. Let's go through them, one by one.

Be Proactive

Stick to the positives. You always want to have positive goals. For example, instead of saying, "I want to stop eating unhealthy snack foods," try setting your goal this way, "I will make healthier snack choices each day." Your goals should inspire you to make positive changes to your lifestyle that promote healthy living, in turn helping you lose the weight. Your goals shouldn't make you feel as though you're being punished. In addition, it's always good for your brain to be fed positive and nurturing thoughts.

Find Meaning in your Goals

Research over the years has shown that people achieve greater satisfaction in life when they work toward things they value, not just goals that bring short-term pleasure or enjoyment. Consciously setting goals that provide positive reinforcement and offer meaning to your long-term desires will ultimately lead to your success. Setting goals or aiming for something that isn't meaningful to you may result in feeling pressured or trapped by something you are not truly committed to, meaning it feels more like a chore than something you really enjoy.

When you tell your mind to stop doing something you will find that is the message that sticks in your head. For example, as soon as you are told not to do something, you immediately want to do it. Has someone ever told you not to do something and then within seconds you find yourself fixated on what you were told not to do?

That's how it works with the brain. To avoid putting yourself in those situations, focus instead on goals that are positive and tell you what to do, not what to avoid doing.

Be Specific and Action-Oriented

In a study by Dr. Faryle Nothwehr and Dr. Jingzhen Yang from the University of Iowa, weight loss was best achieved when the short-term goals were specific to diet or exercise. This indicates that setting those specific goals is an important aspect to getting closer to being thin. What does this mean? People with more than just a goal of getting to a certain weight have better success getting there because they have specific goals working within their desire to lose the weight. Knowing exactly what aspect of diet and/or exercise you are working toward will only benefit you working toward an overarching weight loss goal—whether it's a number on the scale or how you feel in a pair of jeans. Rather than saying "I want to lose weight," try "I will fit into the next size smaller pants." Instead of saying "I want to lose all this excess body fat" (which can sound like a tedious and discouraging task) try "I'm going to lose five pounds over the next month" (which feels far more achievable). Even more action-specific, directly related to your diet, might be a goal related to eating your veggies. Instead of saying, "I want to eat more vegetables," try "I will eat three servings of vegetables a day." Or instead of saying, "I want to eat more fiber," you might say, "This month I will eat two more servings of whole grains each day." Most of the time when you set goals without an action plan, you lose your way.

When it comes to actions and weight loss, you want to be sure that your goals relate to your food intake or physical activity; both of these categories directly impact whether you lose weight, gain weight, or stay at the same weight. By targeting these actions you will be able to set realistic goals that will target your desire to lose weight. By setting goals related to your daily actions, you will take control of your weight, all while making healthy lifestyle changes. These goals also offer your brain a step-by-step guide to your weight loss, which makes success easier to achieve. Plus, as far as your brain is concerned, every success you log—no matter how small—registers as a positive experience, in turn triggering the development of neuronal connections that support more positive achievements in the coming months and years.

If They Can Do It, So Can You

The National Weight Control Registry is a database for an ongoing research study compiling information on how more than 10,000 weight loss maintainers (those who have lost the weight, in this case at least 30 pounds, and kept it off for at least one year) were successful. Looking at the top ways to be successful, 98 percent of the participants changed their food intake habits in some way, while 94 percent increased their daily physical activity. You can see that permanent changes are key to long-term success, and that having goals specific to diet and exercise lays the core foundation for getting yourself thin.

Create a Timeline

Aside from setting up an action plan, nothing is more important than setting up a timeline for your goals. In fact, the action plan and the timeline go hand in hand. This is where organization skills come into play and you really need to focus on what is realistic. Losing large amounts of weight in a short amount of time is not only unhealthy, but also unrealistic, and because of this, setting that as one of your goals can either result in extreme frustration, or possibly worse, regaining that hard lost weight. Dropping weight too rapidly often means when it comes to the long-term timeline, you will have a hard time keeping up with the changes you have made.

Your short-term goals should always support long-term success. This means that making drastic changes just to see quick results will likely backfire because your timeline wasn't realistic. For example, losing 20 pounds in one month is not realistic and therefore not a good (or healthy) goal to set. So, once you have a goal in mind, work on the timeline. "I want to lose two pounds this week." Or, "I will decrease my calorie intake by five-hundred calories every day." Studies have shown that knowing where you're heading with an action and how long you plan to take to get there will double, or even triple, your chances of a successful outcome.

Be a Realist

Confucius said, "Our greatest glory is not in never falling, but in rising every time we fall." When it comes to your body, no one should be more realistic than you, but that doesn't mean you need to beat yourself up when you think about the reality of the current situation. Sure, you may have gained a few pounds over the years, but that shouldn't stop you from making changes now. Being a realist means knowing what your body is capable of and what would be considered healthy for you. You, and only you, can be the judge of what you feel comfortable with. Not considering what is realistic for you can really set you up for big letdowns when it comes time to check back in with your goals. Setting realistic goals with plausible timelines will set you up to be a shining star.

When you initially create your goals, invest some time into breaking them down into smaller pieces complete with a timeline. When it comes to losing weight, most of your goals will be things you will need to stick with long after you reach your weight loss end goal. So the timeline works best by picking a goal—something related to diet changes or physical activity changes—and determining when you want to have fully incorporated that change into your lifestyle. Then just stick with it until it is part of your everyday routine. Once you create that new healthy habit, consider building on that and setting a new short-term goal, getting healthier along the way.

Make sure to account for possible setbacks and have some ideas in place for how to overcome roadblocks. Don't see this as negative thinking but rather as planning for reality. It's always smart to have a Plan B. By doing this, you empower yourself so you and your brain don't feel defeated when those inevitable setbacks occur. Remember, you're only human, and tomorrow is another day. The main desire for everyone—including you!—is really to live a happy and healthy long life.

Monitor Your Progress

Monitoring your progress is the cornerstone of keeping yourself on track for successful goals. Yes, setting a deadline offers you the opportunity to stay on top of what's happening, but recording that progress, either in a journal or similar type of ongoing list, will keep your brain focused on the task. For example, if you set a goal of eating breakfast within one hour of waking up every day, then having a method that will help you check on your progress will keep your brain focused on getting you to commit each morning to starting your day off right by eating something. Set aside time each day, perhaps after meal times, to record your goal-related thoughts, and in no time you will have your brain working hard to remind you each morning to stay on track.

Pay Attention to Your Brain

Now that you have drawn in the attention of your brain, you want to make sure to harness that energy to keep you on track. At the end of each week go back and review your weekly progress to see if you really are on track. Even if you did not entirely meet your goal, when it comes to weight loss, any loss is really a gain.

Perhaps you wanted to eat breakfast every day of the week, but only managed to eat something five of those days. This is where you need to pay attention to your brain. Using the written monitoring of your goals, think about where you hit roadblocks and what you can focus on the next week to help you better reach your breakfast goal. Brainstorming new ways to get to your goal will help you on your journey. Stick with what you're doing and use those new strategies to improve in the coming week, and you will find that you are getting closer and closer to reaching your goal of getting thin.

Reward Your Brain

The last step of the goal-setting process involves self-reward. While these should not be food-related rewards, which would feed your body, aim for motivational rewards, which feed your brain. Think of this as patting yourself on the back. Positive reminders of your success, even if you only met a small goal, will reinforce your intentions and values to your brain, in turn helping to get you to that long-term goal in the distance. For example, letting yourself know that you are proud of yourself and using positive language to reinforce the hard work you have done are good positive ways to remind yourself that you are headed in the right direction. Maybe you passed up a big slice of cheesecake that a friend offered to you at dinner and instead ate a piece of fruit. Telling yourself that you did a good job staying strong with the temptation is a good reminder and motivator to stay on track. At first, you may want to say these things aloud to make sure you're really getting the message.

WHERE'S YOUR FOCUS?

To get thin, you need to find the right things to focus on to maximize your efforts and avoid making mistakes. Here are a few examples of how focus can affect someone on their journey to getting thin:

- If you focus on changing eating habits, your brain will provide new ideas on healthy foods that you can incorporate into your diet. You will better know your likes and dislikes and use this knowledge to your advantage.

- If you focus on learning about good nutrition, your brain will learn to undo the information gathered in attempts at fad dieting or unsafe weight loss practices from the past.
- If you focus on physical activity, your brain will offer up new ideas for what you can do in the gym or at home to burn off more calories each day, and have fun while doing it.

So what are *you* focused on that relates to achieving the weight loss you desire? Have you been focused on the wrong things? If so, it's essential that you work through the steps outlined in this chapter. Chances are, when it comes to weight loss, some of your focus may be misdirected. It's not an easy task, especially if you are focused on a number on the scale. Instead, focus on how you feel.

Bring on Your Insula!

The insula is the part of your cerebral cortex that is associated with emotional processing and empathy. This region can be stimulated in response to something unpleasant. When it comes to thinking about losing weight, there is a good chance you start to feel uncomfortable. Many strong feelings are felt or acknowledged in this region, including gratitude and resentment, both of which are feelings that can be associated with weight loss. There is also research to show this region has a role in addiction, like smoking or drugs, and there is no denying that food can have the same effect on the body, triggering food cravings.

WHY IMMEDIATE GRATIFICATION DEFEATS YOUR PURPOSE

It should come as no surprise that when you set goals in everyday life you will be faced with making the choice between immediate and delayed gratification. When faced with a choice offering a small, immediate reward (losing ten pounds this month) and a larger reward after a delay (losing thirty pounds in six months), research has shown that people will be more likely to choose the smaller, immediate reward over the larger reward further down the road. This habit is referred to as "discounting" by neuroscientists.

In the case of losing weight, instant gratification can put your health at risk and set you up for long-term failure in keeping off the weight. Drastic changes to your eating and exercise habits may result in quick weight loss, but you can't keep up with them for the rest of your life. Instead, focus on setting short-term goals that help you make permanent life changes so you never have the need to seek out instant gratification again with "dieting." Just like in the fable of the tortoise and the hare, "slow and steady wins the race."

HOW YOUR BRAIN BENEFITS FROM INTENTION AND GOAL SETTING

Why not train your brain to function at its top performance level at all times instead of wasting your brainpower by lacking focus. You can do this by looking out for ways to maximize your chances of getting closer to your dreams of looking and feeling great. The more you work on training your brain to be focused on your intentions and goals, the more your brain will work for you. Here are some ways your brain directly benefits from establishing clear intentions and setting realistic goals:

- Intention makes it clear to your brain that what you are doing is true, making it easier for this to happen in real life. Intention also wakes up "sleeping neurons" and strengthens and increases the firing of neural synapses.
- Intention is the foundation for goal setting. This focuses your brain and keeps all the necessary neurons firing.

- Monitoring your intentions will keep your brain focused on the task all day long.
- Rewarding intention reinforces the development of neuronal pathways in your brain. It stimulates your amygdala, in a good way of course, by linking pleasure with goal attainment.

If you train your brain to form new, healthy lifestyle habits, your brain will become accustomed to seeking out and reinforcing those types of rewarding opportunities. The ultimate reward is achieving weight loss and fitting better in your clothes. If you train your brain to focus on what is working, instead of focusing on what isn't, it will begin to recognize far more positives than negatives.

Clearly identifying intention and focusing on the positive things that you are doing for your body will place them front and center in your brain. In return, your brain will bring you new ideas for ways to be happier and thinner—all you have to do is ask.

TIME TO FOCUS ON LEARNING!

Now that you've identified and clarified your intentions, and created goals that will support and foster your weight loss desires, it's time to discuss specific ways you can teach your brain to make solid lifestyle change decisions aimed at getting thin.

CHAPTER 6

LEARN TO GET THIN

Principle: Your brain is still evolving but may respond primitively to modern problems, so you'll have to outsmart it.

Your brain is a fabulous tool that you can use on your path to weight loss success, but your brain also can revert to primitive wiring, resulting in roadblocks along your path. To succeed at getting thin, you need an understanding of the natural way your brain functions, how this could pose some challenges to your intended *get thin* goal, and the steps you can take to prevail over these roadblocks. This chapter will provide you with ways to outsmart and reign in your primitive brain and prevent your instincts from taking over when it could hinder your weight loss efforts.

HANDS OFF THE PANIC BUTTON

Any time you are looking to be successful at something it is natural for fear to take over (that's the amygdala working), but it's important to keep your hands off the panic button. Jumping too often to push that panic button can bring your dreams to a screeching halt. Being unsure or fearful can sabotage any progress you may make at changing your lifestyle and getting thin. To get us started, let's evaluate your comfort level when it comes to a healthy lifestyle.

The *Does "Healthy" Make Me Panic?* Quiz

1. I get my education about diet from:

A. every magazine I read, every news report I hear on TV, and things that my friends tell me.

B. a few websites I like to read daily.

C. my favorite news program.

D. well-respected websites, books, and magazines.

2. When I start a new weight loss plan, I:

A. have no real idea about what I'm doing.

B. do what my closest friends or family members are doing.

C. try listening to cues from my stomach, but don't necessarily pay attention to what I eat.

D. research and evaluate the pros and cons to any changes I may make to my diet.

3. When someone comments on my current weight, I:

A. don't eat for the rest of the day.

B. ask my friends what they think about how I look.

C. start a list of positive things about myself.

D. automatically think about what changes I can make to my lifestyle.

4. When others notice that I have lost some weight, I:

A. immediately think I should eat more because it was too much weight too fast.

B. think I may need to dress in baggier clothes because it's too noticeable.

C. take a peek in the mirror for myself.

D. smile and thank them for their compliment.

5. When I go out to eat, I:

A. order whatever I want so no one notices that I am watching what I eat.

B. order what everyone else is ordering.

C. order what I want, but ask for a to-go box and take some home for later.

D. ask the waiter questions about ingredients and substitutions.

6. When it comes to grocery shopping, I:

A. only go at "off" times so no one sees what I am buying.

B. pick up foods that look healthy, but sometimes I put them back before checking out.

C. read and compare food labels, but sometimes foods I am unsure of end up in my cart.

D. go prepared with a list.

Answer Key

If you picked mostly As, your brain is likely weighted down with fear and it's no wonder you often react rashly or cringe at the thought of making a healthy change. There is no need to blame your brain here because you're the one getting your brain all worked up. This chapter will provide you with a wake-up call and will teach you how to calm your brain and how you can be more rational in the decision making process.

If you picked mostly Bs, you may be impulsive and may find that you tend to stick with the crowd. You must allow your brain to take an occasional break and learn new ways to regulate your decision-making process. Make a few small changes here and there, and your brain will be ready again to take on the role of equal partner.

If you picked mostly Cs, sometimes your brain does really well, firing positively, but you'll find you can make even wiser decisions with a deeper understanding of what needs to be strengthened—and just how easy this is for you to do. Your brain is ready and waiting to be at your service.

If you picked mostly Ds, you are right where you should be, knowing what needs to be done to treat your brain right, and there is a good chance your brain is already serving you—in the form of healthy lifestyle success. Nevertheless, there is always room for improvement, so you will benefit from some minor tweaks to what you are already doing.

POTENTIAL BRAIN PROBLEM AREAS

Nothing is perfect, not even your brain. Even though it can work wonders for you in everyday life, it can also make some crummy decisions. Why? Because your brain may have had no issues dealing with primitive problems, but it can't always stay on top of the crazy, complex society that we're currently living in. Your brain is still expecting threats in the form of large teeth or sharp claws, and a seemingly good way to cope with these threats is to just turn and run, or perhaps stick around and fight it out. Unfortunately, these responses don't work the best when it comes to putting healthy changes in place to help you get rid of some of that pesky excess weight. So, let's identify how your brain's old-world skills can make it hard to function within the new world.

- Your instinctual brain can overtake your more highly developed brain, resulting in letting you make hurried decisions centered on heightened levels of emotion.
- Always looking for the easy way out, your brain will seek out easy ways to come to any conclusion in making a decision, using the least amount of emotion. This habit to take the easy way out can stop your brain from allowing new (and important) information to be included in the decision-making

process, some of which may be helpful when contemplating appropriate lifestyle changes to incorporate in your daily life.

- Your brain's penchant for tree-search processing—limitlessly following thought streams to gather up any and all imaginable data—means you can undoubtedly find yourself lost in thought, and then fail to ever take any action.
- Fear, excitement, and other extreme emotions are highly exciting to your brain. They can be induced by manipulation or perception of the words or actions of others. Emotions can supersede all normal reasoning.
- Your brain can exhibit stubborn behaviors as it becomes set in its ways, resulting in a lack of response when new situations arise.
- You may miss the big picture since your brain has a habit of focusing narrowly on things.
- Immediate rewards may wind up being a setback as your brain may become addicted to them, ranking the pursuit of those rewards (both good and bad) above some of your needs that may really be more important.
- Peer pressure can be a problem since your brain can be overly sensitive to the thoughts and feelings of those around you, making you vulnerable to outside pressure, even though this may hinder your efforts at losing weight. Of course some of this happens at the subconscious level.

The good news is that, during the last 200,000 years, your neocortical brain *has* been evolving to meet and beat the challenges you must overcome in order to survive in the present world. Your brain is flexible, so you have the power to be in control, directing your own thought patterns and teaching your brain how *you* want it to process and interpret your thoughts. Let's not forget one very important piece of information: Your brain is here to serve you!

NOT ONE, BUT TWO BRAINS

Many years ago, well before any modern civilizations developed, humans, just like animals, were forced to rely on instincts. They used their brains for processing sensory information—things like an imminent threat of danger, perhaps a bear lurking in the woods or a drop in air temperature as night approached—and reacted instinctively to this information, usually with a fight-or-flight reaction, like turning and running the other way or finding some way to keep warm during the night. You may have noticed that humans still utilize that instinctual brain every day, and that the information that you get from this can be vital when it comes to making healthy choices. As civilizations developed and turned into more complicated and complex societies, it was imperative that our brains also evolved to keep up with changing demands of everyday living. So, in response, the insightful brain (specifically the PFC) has greatly expanded, both in size and scope, and now plays a key role in processing the complicated social and cultural situations we find ourselves in, including those that involve making decisions about food.

Just be wary, as it is still rather easy for your instinctual brain to take the steering wheel and override your insightful brain, driving you to make hurried decisions rooted in emotions, just as we have had to do historically (think millions of years), in place of making decisions relying on knowledge and logic, which has only become necessary in recent times. Therefore, it's entirely up to you to take notice of the danger this presents to your goals and desires, so that you can take back that steering wheel and allow your insightful brain to be in the driver's seat, not your instinctual one, when making healthy lifestyle decisions.

Let's take a look at the specific ways your two brains can influence you.

Your Instinctual Brain

Just as it sounds, your instinctual brain is the more primitive part of your brain, which is composed of your basal ganglia and limbic system (amygdala and nucleus accumbens); remember these old friends from Chapter 2? Your instinctual brain collects all sensory information (internal and external) and responds instinctively to keep you free from harm. This mechanism and ability to act reflexively is what results in species survival because it responds immediately and appropriately to threats (e.g., those large teeth or big claws). This is the foundation of the fight-or-flight response, which you have probably experienced at least once in your life.

Here are some key attributes of your instinctual brain:

- It accepts and then relays messages from the outside environment, and is responsible for forming your initial "impression" of things happening at any given moment.
- Its focus is primarily on your basic needs—looking for what you need for survival. In this manner, the main focus is on avoiding high-risk situations and looking for other situations that will reward you in your goals.
- It is subjective.
- It is not a fan of uncertainty, and tends to reframe any potential problems until it's easy to understand and act upon them. It leans more toward an all-or-nothing thought pattern.

Now you can see why using just your instinctual brain may inhibit any progress you are making toward losing weight. Listening to this part of your brain may seem like the safe way to go, but those safe choices could be what are holding you back from reaching your weight loss goals.

Your Insightful Brain.

Your insightful brain, also known as your *reflective* brain, is the more developed region, specifically containing your PFC and associated areas. It is responsible for receiving and processing incoming information from your "other brain"—the instinctual brain. It searches through your memory banks for more information, links the situation to relevant memories you have stored, assigns value and rank to each situation, and, if it has the time, weighs all the possibilities before making any decision about what action you should take, if any.

A Primitive Brain Can Be Dangerous in Modern Times

There is no getting around it. Your instinctual brain can naturally jump in and take over. As soon as your limbic system (specifically your amygdala and your thalamus) picks up outside sensory information (sights, sounds, smells), these parts will determine whether that stimulus is "good" or "bad" within a fraction of a second. The first reaction you experience is the instinctual reaction. After this, the message is delivered to your insightful brain (cerebral cortex) that either the situation has been taken care of or that it needs additional assessment since the instinctual part of your brain cannot make conclusions about what a particular external stimulus means in regards to your basic survival. Unfortunately, those initial assessments are embedded in millions of years of evolution and it's possible they are way off base in the situations we encounter in our modern lives. So, you don't want your instinctual brain to rule your decision making, especially in cases where those decisions are related to the complex process of determining where, when, and what to eat.

Here are some key attributes of your insightful brain:

- It receives and processes incoming data from your instinctual brain, then searches through your memory bank for possible connections that can be used in the evaluation process, and allows for the ranking of new information in terms of urgency or value.
- Its focus is on those higher thought processes (e.g. analytical thinking versus just recalling facts) making the most of complex and analytical thinking.
- It plays a role in anticipating what will happen, allowing you to make plans for the future.
- It is predominately objective, using facts to make decisions.

When compared to your instinctual brain, it is easy to see why calling on your insightful brain can better help guide you in making critical judgments about your behaviors, thereby making you healthier and thinner.

How This Applies to Getting Thin

When you are trying to lose weight, you are probably aware—and others have probably told you—that you want avoid relying on your instinctual brain, and instead rely on your insightful brain. This is not always easy to do, especially when your environment sends an emotional trigger (entering the kitchen where someone just baked fresh chocolate chip cookies) or perhaps there is an internal stimulus (you got into a fight with your partner or mother) that results in your instinctual brain kicking in.

This can actually be dangerous when the situation calls for more serious reflection and control before acting, such as in the following situations:

- Deciding what to do when you have a rough day at work.
- Attending a party where dinner is being served.
- Deciding where to go for lunch when you forgot to pack your lunch for work that day.
- Holding back when a coworker brings donuts in to work on a Monday morning.

It's at these times, and in many other similar circumstances, when letting your instinctual brain do the thinking can lead to poor decision-making related to food intake and exercise habits. When you let your instinctual brain take over, and your appetite call the shots, you send yourself down a slippery slope. Keeping that in mind, let's investigate how you can consciously conjure up your more evolved, insightful brain to make healthy lifestyle decisions.

Appetite and Your Instinctual Brain

Appetite is your desire for food that is based on psychological responses to external cues, rather than internal physiological cues in response to hunger. Instinctually, it would make sense that the body would get ready for food just by seeing it or smelling it, especially many years ago when food was scarce, so if it showed up in front of you that meant it was time to refuel—you didn't know when the next mealtime was coming. However, in our modern world, food is rarely scarce, and our appetites may have grown accustomed to delicious delicacies. The overabundance of food can trigger a mindless reaction that lets your instinctive brain call the shots when it sees or smells food that seems appetizing, whether you are truly hungry or not.

GET IN THE DRIVER'S SEAT OF YOUR BRAIN

The process of decision-making results in an imbalance in how your brain functions. Since your brain desires closure, it naturally hunts for the most efficient way to get back to that original state of balance. Additionally, in the event that your brain becomes saturated with stress-related neurochemicals when it can't really spend the time needed for thoughtful and reflective decision-making, it will return to those simpler, instinctive reactions. On the other hand, when you aren't under pressure, it's more likely that you will get the reaction and input you need from your insightful brain. Just as you would expect, as soon as that stress level goes up again, and your insightful brain just isn't responding fast enough, your instinctual brain can kick back in to take care of the job—meaning you are left to rely on emotions rather than on knowledge and objectivity.

This is why you should make sure to take your time when you are faced with important decisions each and every day about what to eat or when to fit in physical activity. Don't rush yourself, and certainly don't let anyone else rush you. For example, if you're in a line ordering food and you notice a line forming behind you simply step off to the side or let someone go in front of you to reduce your own stress level. Activities to reduce stress—including meditation, mindfulness, breathing exercises, positive visualization, mental rehearsal, and thought control (all of which we will discuss in Chapter 8)—will assist your brain to really strengthen that reflective processing of your instinctual brain. You can find a more encompassing list of actions you can take in the Appendix: Specific Things You Can Do to Train Your Brain to Get Thin.

DEFY YOUR BRAIN'S FIXATION ON PATTERNS

Perhaps you've heard the saying "everything happens in threes." There's a good reason as to why we are so quick to believe this, despite having little objective proof that it's true. There is a module, located in your brain's left hemisphere, that is programmed to seek out patterns and make causal relationships and connections, even if there are none present.

Why We Feel Unsettled with Random Occurrences

Randomness is difficult for people. Studies have shown that people really do have a hard time drawing patterns that are truly "random." Let's say we asked that you make random marks down a line. Since your brain is so hard-wired to recognize patterns, you actually have to work really, really hard to make it truly "look random." You would most likely end up creating some form of a pattern, despite your best efforts to resist this habit. Oh, and even if you had been successful at creating a truly random drawing, there's a good chance you would probably think that it resembled a pattern and then alter it, thereby *turning* it into a pattern! It's basically not possible to do this task successfully since our brains don't really even understand random and what this would resemble.

Since this is predominately the task of your instinctual brain, you tend to seek out patterns subconsciously. Then, if you spot a pattern, your brain generally accepts this as fact. For example, when something occurs for the first time (you eat one chocolate chip cookie and then you weigh yourself and find you gained 1 pound), your brain questions if there is perhaps causation ("If I eat another cookie will I gain another pound?"). If you eat another cookie and you do, in fact, gain another pound, your brain tends to react reflexively ("Yes! I was right!"), and the next thing you know, your brain has jumped to what seems to be a logical conclusion ("Eating a cookie makes me gain weight"), thereby connecting the observed pattern to causality. Therefore, in place of an "I wonder" response coming from your insightful brain, you will get an "I know" response coming from your instinctual brain, and in time you have begun to expect what will happen rather than process the information in a thoughtful way—which could unintentionally create a negative relationship with foods.

Identifying patterns and linking them up with past events helped primitive man with survival, and those who had looked for, recognized, and responded to patterns lived to pass their genes on to the next generation. This in turn wired basic survival skills into their instinctual brain, which you have inherited years down the road. Unfortunately, we are always looking for patterns and connections automatically. This is basically now an unconscious reaction, and while you can't flip the off switch, you can learn to spot it when it's happening, and recruit your insightful brain to override this fixation to assign patterns and some meaning to something that is random.

Reduce Unconscious Conformity Bias

Let's face it: survival is a key part of everyday life, so your brain wants to seek out patterns. Predictability in life makes it much more likely that you will survive and, consequently, be able to pass along your genetic material. This is why we are apt to experience something known as "conformity bias," which means that we translate information to conform to those patterns already in place in our brain. For example, keeping with the scenario above, let's say you eat a cookie, but you don't gain any weight at all. Instead of thinking "Oh, maybe I was wrong that eating a cookie makes me gain a pound," you are more likely to conclude, "Well, I must have done some extra exercise today!"

Soften Your Emotional Reactions

As soon as your brain has decided that responses are indeed predictable, it will respond with panic if/when that pattern is not followed, even if there was never a true pattern present. If you react emotionally, your instinctual brain could take control, resulting in unnecessary panic, worry, and even the classic habit of overreacting. In addition, your instinctual brain is so attuned to your routines and habits that when it comes to finding similarities it can spring to attention when it realizes that something is different or out of place. When something like that happens, your instinctive brain can get really riled up and force you to halt the task you are working on and focus your attention instead on whatever it was that caused the panic.

Know that this part of your brain yearns to decode situations and information in an effort to make sense of the surrounding environment. This part believes it can (and will) figure out things in the world. However, a continual hunt for patterns and justifications in random or intricate data can result in subpar decision-making skills—including a decision about what to eat for dinner.

Here are some ways in which you can rein in your instinctual brain when faced with important decisions about leading a healthy lifestyle and getting thin:

- Beware of emotions and the charged language those bring to your brain.
- Don't make a habit of expecting the same results each time you partake in a healthy (or not-so-healthy) practice.
- Monitor and limit exposure to ever-changing information: avoid magazine headlines that draw you in with promises or news reports of a new study (remember, it takes more than one study to change the course of science).
- Look long and hard at all the possible outcomes of your lifestyle changes.
- Stop, take a deep breath. Now, think twice . . . and then a third time.

Bringing yourself back to the moment and processing the information in a logical manner, more than once, will help you make reasonable and doable changes that you can implement and stick with permanently.

GAIN CONTROL OVER TREE-SEARCH PROCESSING

Your brain's abilities are dependent upon its capabilities, and your brain is only as good as its ability to store memories, make connections among information, and understand complex issues. Unfortunately, your brain also has a penchant for tree-search processing: the never-ending flow of thought streams, which gather up all possible and imaginable data, and can ultimately lead to a potentially debilitating inability to make a decision.

Essentially, once your instinctual brain has been given a message and it has been processed, the brain can make connections among packets of information, the neurons divide out (making branches), and link together strongly. When new information comes in and is associated with the previous information, your instinctual brain branches out even further. Now, when the time comes to process new information, your brain feels a need to go searching through all of those branches, so it can find info that it's already processed to match with the new info that's coming, until it is left with no other areas to search.

It's this process that makes some people get caught up in the little details, having their brains scour each and every branch to gather up every little crumb of information—but, in the end, this just weighs down their brain and impedes all their efforts at reaching a resolution. Needless to say, overturning this habit is not an easy process. With a little time and practice, however, it is possible to suppress this instinctual behavior, recognize which information is really relevant in that situation, and get rid of the unnecessary information. To avoid getting lost in information overload, you can train yourself in the technique of mindfulness (covered in Chapter 8), which helps you focus energy and attention toward what's ultimately relevant to that situation.

CAREFULLY EVALUATE RISK

We all possess an intrinsic dislike for the uncertain. This stems from our ancestors and the consequences they faced during life-threatening challenges. If they made the decision to move over to a location that was packed with predators or that experienced little rainfall, the consequences of limited food sources or danger from animals would be present. This level of uncertainty meant their brains continuously stayed on high alert as a result of establishing a low-level constant stream of chemicals promoting this heightened state, in which they experienced fear and needed to rely on a proper response to threats at a moment's notice. Despite not being the best of living conditions, this developed sense of hypersensitivity ensured higher rates of survival.

Why You Have Better Decision Making Power When You Suppress Fear

Your body is armed with a range of chemicals (think powerful weapons), both positive and negative, that will help you get through situations. At times when you are experiencing anger, and especially during times of panic and fear, your limbic system (that instinctual area) will release cortisol, the stress hormone. Cortisol sets off an alarm in your body, telling your regulatory systems that there is a threat, setting off your fight-or-flight response, and ultimately freezing you by stopping your ability to make rational decisions or have any rational thoughts. Conversely, positive experiences and feelings of confidence release serotonin into the body, promoting a feeling of calmness and allowing your brain to slow down and actually think logically through things. So it's up to you . . . which weapon will you choose?

Over the course of history, people who focused on their safety and survival outlived those who didn't, and they were able to pass on those genes that made them avoid risk. Since your brain has a habit of avoiding risk, your instinctual brain may try to take over, stopping you from trying new things and changing old, comfortable habits, even though they may be keeping you from being healthy. Stored fat tissue is a survival mechanism as well, but nowadays many people have excess fat that takes it from being a protective factor (living through a famine later in the year) to a risk factor for chronic diseases like diabetes and high blood pressure. Learning to take on new risks when it comes to getting healthy and allowing your insightful brain to call the shots will help you progress to a thinner, new you.

PUT FEAR BACK IN ITS PLACE

Fear doesn't give you a positive mood or experience. Just hearing about bad news, whether it be a heinous crime, economic issues, or a natural disaster, is enough to cause a person to more than double their estimate of their own chances of risks that aren't even related to the bad news they heard. For example: hearing about a recent string of bank robberies all the way on the other side of the country may lead you to start worrying, out of the blue, about your health, family, or finances. Hearing about bad news puts the idea that bad things can happen in your mind, and you become overly sensitive to all things that remind you of these potential risks—even risks that aren't likely to affect you.

Don't let this fear take over and prevent you from making strong choices about your health. On the other hand, don't let this fear make you rush into creating new healthy habits that aren't well thought out because you may have a hard time sticking with them—and failing to do so may hinder your success in the long run.

The Impact of Fear on Your Brain

When your instinctual brain is scared, fear is placed front and center, which stops your brain from being able accomplish tasks related to critical thinking. Your amygdala, which gets all fired up when fear enters the picture, ignores any other incoming sensory information until you have put an end to whatever triggered the fear in the first place. This really starts to cause problems when you are experiencing fear at an unconscious level. When that happens, you aren't even cognizant of the fact that your PFC has stopped working, which could result in you feeling paralyzed from all the anxiety you're experiencing. You may lose all concentration and may not be able to focus on what seems to be just a simple, everyday task. Instead, your brain is on overdrive, scanning around for the root of your fear or any other threat present in your environment. Basically, your instinctual, primitive brain is placed on high alert, while your insightful, thinking brain is pushed into the back seat. It's hard to want to be healthy if you are frozen in fear.

Why You Might Want to Wait Before Eating That Food

Looking at the research, studies demonstrate that around 50 percent of people are able to recognize when bad news has disturbed them in some way. However, only 3 percent of people will actually admit that being shaken up over that news may impact their reactions to other risks. The evidence points to the idea that we definitely experience an impact when it comes to hearing bad news. If you've just gotten some bad news, make sure to wait before making any decisions, especially decisions related to eating. You'll want to wait until your emotions have calmed down and there are fewer of those stress chemicals floating around. Your body will thank you for it later.

How to Silence Your Amygdala

Since the amygdala focuses on fear, it is important to silence it when it comes to decision-making. There are a few ways to go about this, including visualization, meditation, mental rehearsal, relabeling, and creating a soothing, loving-kindness mantra, discussed below and in later chapters. By being able to acknowledge when you are fearful or when you are in situations that could cause fear, even unconsciously, you are able to silence an overactive amygdala. Your anticipation of fearful situations and visualizing positive outcomes, whether through visualization, mental rehearsal, or meditation, will provide the neural foundation that your brain needs in order to know what steps to take when fear and panic sets in.

This is how it works:

- When you use **visualization**, the technique of picturing something in your mind, neuronal pathways are created that can counteract visceral neuronal rut, assisting in making sure that similar (even vaguely similar) future situations come out more smoothly.
- **Mental rehearsal**, the technique of practicing an event or activity in your mind to help you improve a skill, (covered in Chapter 7) helps you feel prepared for whatever situation may be placed in front of you, increases your confidence level, and works to place a strong neuronal foundation, which is necessary for you to become successful.
- **Meditation**, a trained practice of concentration to help you focus your energy and mind, (covered in Chapter 8) brings you to a more aware state, increasing your ability to notice fears as they pop up, and helps to keep your emotions in control.
- **Relabeling**, or giving a new name to a situation can impact how you will respond emotionally. When faced with what you would think of as a "problem," you might start to feel a bit

overwhelmed given the circumstances. However, if you relabel (or call) this a "challenge" instead of a "problem" you in turn summon up your competitive nature and soon you will be ready to take on that challenge headfirst.

- **Loving-kindness** (or self-compassionate) meditation establishes positive emotions and, in stressful situations, will have a calming effect on your amygdala.

Utilizing these techniques helps you get a grasp on the present situation and gives you the ability to better handle future situations that relate to making choices that impact your health and wellness, and weight.

Don't Act Scared

People who experience success (no matter what the situation) tend to avoid fear and fearful responses and instead focus on using their brains to find new, creative solutions to their problems. They don't wallow in pessimism. Instead, they work on problem solving, exercising their minds, and finding ways to overcome challenges.

It is possible, believe it or not, to rewire your brain and have it stop reacting to situations purely based on fear. Fear hides in places you may not even realize, which could be preventing you from taking that next step to losing weight. Maybe you are afraid of the hard work or unsure of what will happen when you shed the pounds, but there are many possibilities when it comes to the fear of finally taking control of your life. Fear triggers a typical and instinctual response. In order to offset this early reaction, you need to scrutinize exactly what is at the root of your fear. Latching on to your insightful brain's resources you can wiggle out from under your usual, fear-based responses and use the available evidence to make decisions.

BEWARE OF GETTING CAUGHT IN NEURONAL RUTS

As we've previously discussed in this chapter, your brain tends to get set in its ways, often responding in a very programmed way when placed in new situations. Never doubt the power of fear. It can heighten your sensitivity in those new situations, and make matters worse by releasing stress hormones; it ultimately stops any ideas that you may have before your intellectual brain has a chance to consider them. Then you run the risk of entering a full-blown panic, and any wish for new and creative solutions to your problems will crumble beneath the outpouring of emotions. To make matters worse, your basal ganglia have the ability to "remember" past bouts of panic. When your basal ganglia become overactive, they are more reactive to stress hormones, including cortisol, meaning it will take less cortisol in each subsequent occurrence of panic for you to jump right into that fight-or-flight status. As a result, it becomes difficult for you to take risks, even if they are not seemingly risky. For example, these stress hormones may make it hard for you to cook a healthy meal for your family if you're not sure they'll like it, or fit in a weekend workout at the gym if you're worried about how you look in your gym clothes.

Should you find yourself stuck in a rut of fear or panic, find a new and interesting (or possibly even risky) situation to take part in to help you learn to beat your fears and retrain your working memory to place a focus on the specific facts, rather than the emotional response you have attached to them. If you find that you are still trapped in the clutches of fear, practice calming methods (like deep breathing, labeling your fears, challenging assumptions) as you wait until you have a better handle on the situation and can see things more positively.

In time, with concentrated attention—and, of course, dedicated practice—your brain will sail right over those neuronal ruts, making it easier for you to get a grasp on your fear, put it in perspective, and employ your insightful PFC at the precise moment that it is needed for critical evaluation.

Understand the Limitations of Your Working Memory

The part of your memory that is focused on the here and now is your working memory—the seven or so chunks of data, whether it be words or numbers, that easily stay in your mind at any one time for about 20–30 seconds. It can be so in tune with what's happening right then and there, looking for all immediate solutions or similar processes, that your brain never gets the chance to be thrust into gear and let you maintain a rational thought. Here's a little about how your memory operates, plus a little on its limitations:

- Your short-term memory is preoccupied with the immediate happenings in your life, and it is still processing information to decide if any of it is worth remembering.
- Your long-term memory contains those pieces of information that you've decided to hold on to for longer than five minutes and tasks your brain with filing this information and linking it with things that are similar.
- Your working memory holds on to the few facts that you are keeping in your mind from moment to moment, and is placed on lockdown until you have spent time dealing with the fearful emotions you may be experiencing in that moment, so it cannot register any other information, like calming cues.
- Tying your basal ganglia up dealing with responses to fear and panic, and allowing your brain to be flooded with cortisol, prevents your insightful brain from finding better solutions.

Gaining an understanding of the limitations of your memory will allow you to give your working memory the space and time needed to support you in a variety of situations, and will even help you focus on remembering just the facts you need to successfully manage your weight.

TEACH YOUR BRAIN TO STOP MAKING THE SAME OLD MISTAKES

As you know, your brain has a habit of seeking predictable patterns, so it makes sense that you may catch yourself making the same diet and exercise mistakes time and time again. Unfortunately, this only makes it harder for you to be successful at losing weight and keeping it off. You could even say that your brain prefers predictability over new and changing actions—even if those same old decisions give you negative results!

Don't fall victim to this. Instead, fight it with all your might! To do this you need to make your brain consciously aware of these mistakes. From time to time, make a list of all the mistakes you make when trying to change your lifestyle to include more healthy habits. Now, ask yourself: "What are the negative diet and exercise habits I had that were hindering my ability to lose weight?" These could include mistakes like the following:

- Not planning meals/snacks in advance
- Being quick to make food-related decisions
- Rationalizing not going to the gym
- Letting fear rule your choices
- Ignoring that your weight was a problem
- Eating in emotional response to problems
- Being afraid to cook more fresh meals at home

Although the items on your list may vary from these, this list will be helpful in taking the next step. Now that you have your list, consciously decide on an action plan that will help you learn from those mistakes and strengthen your ability to lose weight in the future.

READY, SET, FOCUS

Whatever has *your* focus will become the focus of your brain. You can train your brain to think positive, effective, and success-driven thoughts, or you can do the opposite and teach it to focus on fear and negativity. The second choice will stick you right where you don't want to be, which is right where you are—or at an even higher weight. It really does make a difference what you lead your brain to focus on and how you decide to react. You control your mind, so you can pick what to focus on: the positive or the negative. Will you test the boundaries of your brain? If you don't, it may respond by falling into those same old neuronal ruts, keeping you focused on the negative instead of opening up new neuronal pathways that allow you to move forward and make healthy lifestyle changes.

As Far as the Eye Can See

Think about what you see out there on the horizon. Is it a new, thinner you? It should be! Look out as far as the eye can see. This newer version of you may be months down the road, and, in fact, it shouldn't be just around the corner. Many times fear will kick in, and months away *does* sound like a long time, but changing habits takes time, too. In fact, it will take different amounts of time for everyone, so don't judge your progress on that of others. Otherwise you are likely to bring on those panicked moments and fear (along with your instinctual brain) will kick into overdrive.

You want to be using your insightful brain to process the information needed to make decisions about changing your daily habits, aiming for small changes that are reasonable to incorporate into each and every day. By using your insightful brain, you are better able to focus on the long-term results. To help ensure that your brain remains focused on the long view and isn't prone to chasing short-term (and short-lived) gratification, try these techniques:

- Create a personal healthy lifestyle plan that includes both your short-term and long-term goals.
- Base your weight loss and exercise decisions on what is likely to benefit you more over the long term.
- Don't measure your weight loss (in pounds per week or month) against others since everyone will be different. Doing this may force you to want to lose more weight faster even if it isn't the best for the long term.
- Don't weigh yourself every day.
- Reevaluate your goals and lifestyle choices (healthy or not-so-healthy habits) every couple of months.

Look Out for Addictive Tendencies

It's only natural to feel a rush when you notice that you have lost weight or your body has changed shape (for example, you fit into those pants that you couldn't wear the week before), but this can feel so good to you that your brain seeks out opportunities, almost compulsively, to recreate the that rush. This can result in negative relationships with food and negative behaviors when it comes to getting healthy. The joy of seeing the number on the scale go down can result in a desire to lose more weight in a shorter amount of time, resulting in unhealthy practices to lose the weight. Remember, overtraining, such as running too many miles too soon, or exercising in the gym twice a day or for multiple hours at time, can injure your body and even stunt your weight loss because it puts stress on your body and triggers the flight-or-fight response.

It is important to remember that while it may sound easy to make a few changes, it really takes discipline to stick with lifestyle changes and not get distracted by the many temptations lurking at every turn.

CAUTION, CAUTION! AVOID HERD MENTALITY

Humans are vulnerable to something known as herd mentality. This is when you pick up verbal and/or visual cues from the people around you. Basically, you tend to follow the pack, or "go with the flow." Sure, everyone else may be doing it, but that doesn't mean it's positive or good for you. You jump right in without weighing the consequences and thinking for a moment before making a thoughtful, informed decision. Maybe we don't live in herds or tribes anymore, but the innate behavior is still buried inside of us. If you want to lose weight and keep it off, falling prey to herd mentality will only slow you down.

It might sound good to hear about how a new diet promises to help you lose the weight without changing your diet, that there are new super foods that will help melt off the pounds, or that there is a miracle cure for obesity—unfortunately, these promises just don't pan out. The problem is that so many people will try them and you will start to hear success stories. Any time someone is focused on watching what they eat and getting into a new exercise plan they will naturally be more in tune with what they are eating (and likely the diet is *forcing* some kind of food restriction) and no matter what the diet plan includes or excludes, the person will lose weight. At first there is water weight shed, but that is coupled with an unavoidable reduction in calories, and any reduction in calories, not just from foods on a "magic" list, results in weight loss—especially soon after starting. So, it may sound like this "diet" is working for everyone, and it may actually *be* working in the short term, but if your goal is long-term weight loss success, following the latest, trendiest "diets" will only get you as far as the next new plan you hear about, and you won't have a lot to show for it.

SO, WHAT DOES IT ALL MEAN?

We have given you a lot of information so far, and there is more to come, so while you don't have to commit every tidbit we share to memory, you will be significantly more successful in reaching your *thin* goals if you have an understanding of how your brain works. You will also gain a greater appreciation for the differences between your instinctual and insightful brain and how each can really affect your daily healthy lifestyle decisions. It is key for both parts to work harmoniously, balancing emotions with critical thinking, in order to be able to evaluate your options and then make thoughtful, informed decisions. Just don't forget that your instinctual brain will be quick to respond to any emotional messages sent to the brain, and it is always easier to follow with instinct rather than power up and engage your insightful, analytical brain.

As we will cover in the following chapter, there are specific actions you can take to repress your instinctual brain and strengthen the capabilities of your insightful brain. So let's get to work!

CHAPTER 7

WORK HARD TO GET THIN

Principle: Your brain is capable of growing in harmony with your needs, and is also stimulated as a result of your actions.

You've learned many different facts about your brain so far in this book, but in this chapter you'll get more info about your brain's laziness factor. You may think that you're the one who's lazy if you miss a workout or don't get up much during the day, but if your brain was left to its own devices, it would always seek the easy way out and you will always get the easiest solution to your problem or situation. However, the easy way out is generally the solution that your quick-to-respond instinctual brain produces, which means that your conclusions tend to be driven by your emotions, and not so much by the important information at your disposal. The previous chapter discussed how you can make more rational decisions based on logic. By learning to silence your quick responses based on fear or panic, you will be better able to let your insightful brain do the work, using facts to come to your conclusions.

Now, you can take this one step further and learn to engage your PFC more frequently, training your insightful brain to put its resources to work and have you thinking longer and harder. This skill will help you make wise decisions when it comes to daily habits that work to keep you hidden under the excess fat or help you to shed the excess weight and get yourself thin. To do this you will have to build up the neuronal pathways of your insightful brain, focusing on reason rather than letting your instinctual brain be your crutch for making important, healthy decisions.

DON'T STRAIN YOUR BRAIN

It's not uncommon in today's busy world for your brain to get bogged down, overtaxed, and utterly strained, but some people overload their brains more than others. Take this quiz to see how you're doing.

The *Am I Straining My Brain?* Quiz

1. **With multitasking, I:**

   A. have no problem managing around five things at the same time.

   B. can handle about two or three things at once, but that's about it.

   C. know I'm in too deep when I'm working on two things at the same time.

   D. never multitask when I'm focused on something of importance.

2. **I review all incoming e-mails, texts, and messages:**

   A. immediately.

   B. about once an hour.

   C. five or so times daily.

   D. only once or twice a day.

3. **When I am deciding what to order at a restaurant, I:**

   A. barely have a chance to look at the menu since I am checking messages and engaging in conversation.

   B. spend a few minutes looking at the pictures on the menu while I am also looking at messages on my phone or talking to friends.

   C. review the menu, but sometimes get easily distracted.

   D. focus on the menu and look for healthier items to choose from.

4. **When I go grocery shopping, I:**

   A. am usually in a hurry, answer my phone at least once, and forget some of the items I needed.

   B. am sometimes in a hurry and occasionally stray from what I need because something catches my attention or I get a craving for a certain food.

   C. take a list of needed items, but may pick up a few other items if a sale catches my attention or I see someone buy something that looks good.

   D. go when I have list of items I need and I stick to the list.

5. **When I am at work, I:**

   A. am working on many tasks at once and worrying about what I need to do at home.

   B. Pick two or three major tasks to work on, and occasionally think about things I need to do at home, like cook dinner.

   C. spend most of my time focused on one task, and will also think about what needs to be done at home, like cook dinner.

   D. focus just on the important task for the day related to my job.

6. **During exercise, I:**

   A. think about all the things I should be doing instead because I may not have enough time later in the day.

   B. think about a variety of things and brainstorm ideas for work and personal life activities.

   C. listen to music, watch TV, or read a magazine.

   D. clear my mind and focus on my movements.

Answer Key

If you checked mostly As, you simply aren't allowing your brain a fair chance at firing up. As a result you may find yourself struggling to make it through the day. You have become the victim of information overload, which has overstimulated and overtaxed your brain. Your emotional responses and inefficiency at responding based on facts can be significantly improved, but you need to give your brain the chance to do this.

If you checked mostly Bs, there are a lot of things going on concurrently and, yes, your brain does feel the strain. You will find that your brain, and ultimately you, will function at a higher level once you have your daily life tasks under control. Then you can put your brain to its best use.

If you checked mostly Cs, while you seem to be coping pretty well with everyday life and don't feel too overwhelmed, in reality, you still have too much going on at once. Your need to be looking out for your brain and making sure you are giving it ample time and space to allow you to be successful.

If you checked mostly Ds, you have a good grip on your priorities and are well-versed in managing your daily tasks. As always, there is room for improvement, so with careful attention paid to your brain, you'll discover that you can make wiser decisions, taking your success at creating a healthy lifestyle one step ahead of where you are now.

MULTITASKING MISTAKE

You can't deny that you live in a world where multitasking (or least attempting to multitask) is the norm. Everyone is doing something, while doing something, while doing something else. Unfortunately, your brain is designed to focus its attention on whichever single task it considers to be the most important. Somewhere in the course of history, humans decided to shift from doing one task at a time to doing multiple things at once. Sometimes you may even find that you are trying to do upward of ten different things at once, although this usually produces horrible results (example—talking on a cell phone while driving).

The plain and simple truth is that your brain is just not, at any time, able to focus on more than one task. Technically, you are not really multitasking even if you think you are, because your brain will really be switching between tasks—you can never give two (or more) tasks 100 percent attention or focus at the same time. So, for example, when you take a phone call and are talking while driving, you only think that you're giving your attention to both tasks. In reality, you're not. Your brain could be focused on the driving, but as soon as the person on the phone says something that requires a reply, your brain switches back over to the conversation and switches your focus off the driving entirely.

The more tasks you take on at one time, the less efficient your brain becomes; it's also far less likely to focus on the most important task, which means that it is no surprise that people using their phones while driving have car accidents. Multitasking will also increase the energy demands placed on your brain, which results in feeling worn down later on. This is precisely why it's a good idea to remove as many distractions as you can when you are trying to complete a task that needs your undivided attention, like at meal or snack times. Distractions will ultimately lead you to poor food choices and can even result in mindless eating—that's right, you may never even notice what you have been eating!

INFORMATION OVERLOAD

If you ever felt like you couldn't make a decision because there were just too many options or pieces of information, then it's likely that you have fallen victim to information overload. For example, maybe you have been given so much information about what kinds of exercises to do that you still don't know what exercises are right for you. Information is tossed at us daily from just about every direction. It's no surprise that there is research currently going on to look at what happens when you are given too much information—something popularly referred to as "analysis paralysis." This condition of feeling like you have way too much information to address has become so commonplace that an entry was added in 2009 to the *Oxford English Dictionary* for "information fatigue." While the concept is not new, the realization that information overload does more than just leave people feeling drained and frustrated, and that it really hinders cognitive function, is relatively new. There is recent research regarding the science of decision-making that shows how too much information leads people to make poorer choices, often ones they regret later on. You can see why information overload coming from food advertisements, or even restaurant menus, may ultimately lead you to make a poor decision when it comes to eating habits.

All the info that comes into your brain will offer three possible options for making a choice: will you reply immediately, will you factor it into a future decision, or will you get rid of it altogether? As you already learned, your working memory holds, at most, seven small pieces of information at any one time. From there, information important enough to hold onto will need to be carried off to your long-term memory, which is an act that requires a conscious effort on your part. While there is still incoming information piling up, your brain starts to struggle with determining what it needs to keep for the future and what can be tossed out. Not paying attention to repetitive incoming information and processing what you won't need for later puts a hold on your cognitive resources. The more information that gets pushed in, the harder it will be for your brain to do its job. Let's take a look at some specific information overload repercussions.

It Affects Your Decision Making

With the onslaught of information shoveled into our brains each day, we are constantly asking our brains to respond on the spot. Even at the expense of making a bad decision, your brain will try to keep up with the demand. If your brain is constantly receiving new information for processing, it typically favors the fast response over the best response.

It Messes with Your Priorities

The natural wiring of your brain is to recognize and then respond to change, which means that any incoming information places a demand on your decision-making brain to start working right away. This is because your brain tends to assume that the most recent, up-to-date news is also the most important. Behavioral economist George Lowenstein of Carnegie Mellon University calls this phenomenon of focusing more on the recent information and overlooking earlier information the "urgency effect." Your brain tends to favor immediacy and quantity over quality.

It Smothers Your Brain's True Brilliance

If you allow yourself to be inundated by a flood of information, you're less likely to make wise decisions throughout the day. You need to give your brain ample time to weave new information into existing information on a subconscious level, and then make new connections as appropriate. You can get tired just thinking about all the work it takes to process the information that's tossed at you daily, but you can give your brain a rest by:

- Placing limits on the incoming information flow. Give it a try—unplug from technology by turning off your television, the Internet, your cell phone, and any other information that gets to you with the touch of a finger.
- Set priorities. This is especially helpful when you are working on something that requires your full attention. You can't make it through the workday and stay healthy, both physically and mentally, if you aren't able to provide those projects with your full attention.
- Be wise in selecting your sources. With all the misinformation out there related to food, nutrition, exercise, and health, make sure to

look at a variety of sources, critically evaluate where the information is coming from, focus on what you consider to be the most reliable/credible sources, and then forget about the others.

- Don't jump right to the conscious process of weighing pros and cons (or whatever similar method you use) when bombarded with complicated information. First allow your unconscious brain the chance to think about it.
- Determine what you consider the most important information needed for each decision, and then focus specifically on those elements instead of every single piece of incoming information. Don't forget that you shouldn't rank information based on when it was received.

By taking these steps to minimize information overload you will find it easier to make important decisions daily.

GRAB THE ATTENTION OF YOUR INSIGHTFUL BRAIN

An easy way to grab the attention of your insightful brain and kick it into high gear is by searching harder to locate evidence to show that something is false rather than focusing on searching for evidence to support that it is true. The nature of your instinctual brain is to avoid uncertainty, so this technique helps you to reshape problems into easy-to-understand terms, like easily classified "truths" that are likely not going to be true in normal circumstances. In order to ensure that you are making smart decisions related to a healthy lifestyle, you need to have your insightful brain counteract those emotional reactions that happen when you fall into instinctual methods of response in situations, whether they are related to a food choice or a decision of where or when to exercise. When you place your focus on proving something *false*, or at least think of some ways that it *could* be false, you grab the attention of your insightful PFC, and allow it to utilize all of its evaluative talents.

For example: If you visited a store that offered you a special "diet" pill that claims proven efficiency at helping others lose weight—a claim backed up by the pictures on the bottle—your instincts may tell you this sounds like a good product to help you lose the weight. The exciting claims may be just enough to get your instinctual brain to eagerly tell you to buy the product. However, the claims just state that this product worked for the person on the label and results may not be typical for others, so there is nothing there that says you will lose the weight too.

To put in its fair share, your insightful brain wants more factual information about the product, the contents, and what else the person did during the time they were taking this *magic* pill. However, even though you have that information, your main question of whether the product really works is still unanswered.

Your instinctual brain might be impressed with the product, but given some time to think about things, your insightful brain is way more likely to recognize that there is no such thing as a *magic* pill or something of a *miracle* product to help you instantly lose weight, and even if it exists, it may not be safe and will likely not produce long-term results. When it comes to losing weight, you really want to make sure you are keeping it off . . . not just losing it temporarily.

HOW TO GET YOUR PFC TO STEP IT UP

The best thing you can do to make sure you make good decisions in situations where you don't have a lot of time to think about it is to have your insightful PFC step up. Asking a lot of follow-up questions (regardless of how silly they may seem) is one easy way to call upon your insightful brain. If you are in a situation where you don't understand the information you are told—either by a personal trainer, a gym employee, dietitian, or anyone else giving you health-related information—take a moment to ask them to explain what this means in simpler terms. Until you are able to "teach" the information back to that person, you are still learning that information. When it comes to your health and understanding of it, it's very true that there is no such thing as a dumb question.

When you are meeting with someone who is giving you important information that will have an impact on your healthy lifestyle decisions and subsequent habits, make sure you have at least three related questions to ask this person. Being prepared will ensure that you get the information that your brain needs to make an informed decision. When it comes to nutrition- and health-related advice, there is a lot of false or misleading information out there. You must weigh the information to make sure you are basing your decisions on the correct information and that you understand exactly what you need to do to incorporate that habit into your daily routine. Don't just take everything at face value, and always remember that with nutrition-, fitness-, and health-related information, everything should be individualized; a one-size-fits-all approach rarely works. Of course, there are many other ways to have your insightful PFC step it up at times when you need to make decisions. These include the following tactics.

Silence Your Emotions

You don't want to ignore your emotions. Instead, recognize and then find ways to silence them so that your brain has *quiet* time while processing relevant information. You may want to take deep breaths, or it may be as easy as recognizing them and bringing rational thoughts to the emotional side, letting those emotions know you hear their concerns and will address them. You may have to distract your emotions and come back to address those (and your fear) at a later time.

Take a Step Back from Your Emotions

Distancing yourself can be a good tool to help you separate yourself from your emotions. Imagine that this is a decision you are making for someone else. How would you counsel them to act in this situation? Thinking you have some "responsibility" for the outcomes of someone else will likely send a wake up call to your insightful brain and bring it to action.

Think Harder

Don't just settle on the first decision that you come to in a situation. Think harder about the outcomes and the options you have, even if it is something that seems as small as deciding what to eat for lunch. While this is a decision that is best made in advance—the night before, if possible—sometimes things come up and that decision needs to be made as lunch hour rolls around. Don't just go with what seems like the best idea because it is the only idea you think you have. There will always be other alternatives and options, so remember that your brain will always seek the easy way out and tends to go with the fastest solution. By not fully bringing your insightful brain into the game, you are likely to end up with instinctual decision-making patterns, possibly even allowing fear to guide your decision. Thinking harder—and longer—about the situation will help you to come to healthier decisions in the end.

Don't Be Fooled

Things are rarely what they seem on the outside—even food products, menu items, gym plans, "diet" guides, and specialty health products. Just because something looks healthy doesn't mean that it is. There is a term in the field, *health halo*, also known as the *halo effect*, which simply means that the appearance or perception of a word or certain look to an item gives people a false sense of belief that it is indeed good for them or "healthy." Don't be fooled by claims that have no definition or meaning when it comes to your health or nutritional status, such as "all natural" or "made with whole grains" (it may have whole grains, but only a very small amount). In many of these cases, there is no true definition or meaning for the claim, but seeing it on a label gives the impression that the food is good for you. In fact, this product may not be healthy at all (although it is possible it may still fit in a healthy balanced diet). Examples of these unhealthy "health" foods include low-fat or fat-free desserts loaded with sugar, fruits canned in syrup, and juices packed with empty calories and added sugar. Call upon your insightful brain to help avoid being fooled by seemingly healthy products that may be sabotaging your weight loss success.

Take a Time-Out

There is no need to make a rash decision about anything during your day that impacts your health and well-being, either positively or negatively. Make sure to take a time-out and really think things through. You need that extra time to let your insightful brain take over and think about things rationally and based on fact. For example, you are asked by some friends from your gym to join them in a high-intensity workout class that meets twice a week. Instead of jumping right into this and saying yes, you need to consider if this is something that is beyond your abilities at this time or something you think you can do without risking injury from pushing yourself too far. Certainly exercise is a positive thing, but pushing yourself beyond your limits can be dangerous and can result in an injury, which in turn could put the brakes on your future workout efforts as you work to recover. Taking a time out and getting back to your workout buddies later will give you some time to rationally weigh the options. We usually like to think that if people we know can do it, so can we (face it, humans tend to be competitive, even if just a little bit), but it is important to remember that everyone has different skill levels and capabilities when it comes to physical activity so it is important to always consider this.

Collect More Information

Make sure you have collected as much of the information that is relevant to your situation as you can. The more information you nourish your brain with, the better able your insightful brain is to respond appropriately. You may not find everything that you need, but since you shouldn't be taking things at face value, you will want to at least find information to support or refute those claims. Not finding out more information can lead not only to poor decision-making, but to potentially dangerous decisions as well. For example, let's say that you have just read a magazine article claiming that a new supplement on the market has been helping people to lose weight quickly. This sounds like a very attractive promise, but before spending money on miracle products you should investigate this more. Since anything you ingest (food or pills) can impact your health, always turn your critical brain on and do some research. If you don't find anything unbiased that supports the claims, then it may be safe to assume it doesn't exist and you should probably pass. Information is key to getting healthy and staying healthy.

Walk It Off

Walking is a double whammy! Not only does this give you a chance to let your mind rest, take a break from the decision-making process, and come back with a fresh perspective, but it also really helps you physically on your quest to get thin. Exercise, not just walking, provides benefits to both your brain and your body, so this will always be a win-win.

Sleep on It

Not all health and wellness, diet, and exercise decisions can be put off until the next day, but there are some that can. While you don't want to wait until tomorrow to decide what to cook tonight for dinner, deciding what gym membership to pick or what exercise program to start may be better left until you have had a good night's sleep. Of course this means that you should take just one good night's sleep to think things over, not that you should keep putting off those decisions until you ultimately take no action at all. Chapter

11 will provide more information about how important sleep can be to your brain and why this age-old saying of "sleep on it" really is good advice, particularly for major life decisions. These may not be directly related to getting thin and lifestyle habits, but they can certainly impact your healthy lifestyle decisions indirectly. Sleep can have positive effects and, just like exercise, will also create a win-win situation since adequate sleep is necessary for maintaining a healthy weight and preventing stress hormones from rising.

Ask Some Questions

When making decisions about healthy lifestyle changes you can make to help you get thin, here are some questions to ask yourself in order to engage your insightful brain and help better evaluate the situation:

- Is this change going to produce positive results for my health?
- Will this habit be harmful to my health?
- How can I make the time each day to be successful in this new habit?
- How much will this cost?
- Is this a feasible change?
- Why am I doing this?
- Can I implement this change for my whole family?
- Is this just a quick fix?
- Will I be able to stick with this in the long run?
- Will my family be supportive of this change/new habit?

By thinking over these questions before implementing new, daily routines and habits into your life, and possibly that of your family, you give your PFC and insightful brain the chance to think the decisions out and not base your actions solely on emotions.

Decisions and Your Brain

To improve your decision-making skills, you can improve those brain functions that are specifically tied to that task. For example, being able to focus helps you make sound decisions because you need to be able to concentrate on the task at hand and the facts you need to make that decision, so any thing you do to improve your focus, no matter what task you are focused on (even something as simple as brushing your teeth), will eventually lead to an improvement in your decision-making capabilities. The good news is that your brain's skills are interchangeable, so developing that skill in one aspect of your life can strengthen it to be applied to other aspects. The following are the chief brain functions associated with decision-making. Think about what you can do to bulk them up.

- **Focus:** Your ability to tune out distractions and focus on the task at hand affects how well you retain information.
- **Control your thoughts:** Your ability to filter and control flow of information in and out of your brain can have an effect on how well you think.
- **Process new information:** Your ability to understand new information will affect your decision making skills.
- **Integrate information:** Your ability to make connections between what you already know and newly gained information affects the amount of information accessible to your thought process.
- **Short-term memory:** Your ability to hold on to any new information learned may affect your decision-making practices, especially if you routinely need to take in a lot of information and make quick decisions.
- **Long-term memory:** Your ability to recall past events that impacted how you look or feel about your weight, both positive and negative, can affect your decision-making as a result of how much emotion is connected to those experiences.

- **Develop new skills:** Your ability to keep your brain firing, active, and plastic will keep it agile and affect how easy it will be to develop new skills.

Nutrition Misinformation Overload

Between the *health halo* effect, perceptions of food products, celebrity diet fads, and magazine articles, it's no wonder that consumers are confused over what to buy and what to believe—or practice! There is a *ton* of information out there about food and nutrition, and not all of this is correct. Letting your brain get overloaded with misinformation will only provide further setbacks when trying to lose weight. Research consistently shows that foods having the appearance of being healthy leads consumers to underestimate the actual calorie content and tends to result in overeating those foods. Flooding your brain with this misinformation and not taking the time to critically think about it does have the power to influence your nutrition decisions. You may think you made a healthy decision, but you could be eating a lot more than you realize, ingesting empty calories, or bloating yourself with extra salt.

Up to this point you've learned—and will continue to learn—ways that you can work to improve how well your brain operates. However, it is entirely up to you to support this learning and put the ideas and recommendations into everyday practice to make sure that your brain is doing everything it can to get to your healthy, thin self. Hard work pays off; in the case of losing weight, that hard work will bring you a lifetime of positive results.

MAKE IT A HABIT TO WORK HARD

Getting your weight under control is no easy task. Like all major accomplishments in life, it takes hard work. If it were easy, we wouldn't have the obesity epidemic that we are facing at this time. If you've tried to lose weight in the past and it seemed easy, there is a very good chance that the weight didn't stay off; perhaps you even gained more back than you lost in the first place. There really is no easy way out, but you can make it easier if you bring your brain into the weight loss equation and train it to help you shed those extra pounds.

In order to get thin, you need to develop a healthy lifestyle, with actions you take daily that impact your energy intake and energy expenditure. To do this, you need to make it a habit to wholly engage your mind and challenge it in all tasks, not just those related to making healthy lifestyle decisions. The more you engage your brain, the better able you are to use it to your advantage when the time comes to make it count for losing the weight. Lazy brains, just like lazy bodies, aren't as likely to be ready to spring into action when you need them. With every use of your brain, the sharper it will become. Every time you introduce new information, or use your complex thinking skills, you strengthen existing synapses and may even form new synapses. You really can reshape your brain just by completing those desired healthy lifestyle tasks on a regular basis, pushing yourself—and your brain—just a little further each time. Keep your brain challenged daily by doing the following:

- Brainstorm ideas for new ways to do the same old tasks.
- Every once in a while, try taking on a project that is outside your comfort zone.
- Learn a new component to the job you already do. Push yourself to learn more about your work and advance yourself in the

office or school. Positive aspects anywhere in your life can spill over into success with managing your weight.
- Learn something entirely new—something that will really challenge you.

It's also important to keep in mind that the less often you do something, the less important your brain will see that action. When you stop working the parts of your brain assigned to certain tasks, you will slowly—but eventually—lose those synapses. Not all hope is lost, though, because much like relearning to ride a bike, those synapses can be reactivated—and it is an easier process than having to learn a whole new task.

Do What the Thin Do

Weight loss maintainers remain aware and conscious of the steps they need to take to keep the weight off. Not only were these thin people successful at losing the weight, but also they remained successful by keeping it off. Looking at the data from the National Weight Control Registry, which tracks the information on more than 10,000 successful weight loss maintainers, the steps those people take each day to keep it off show that they are focused on staying healthy, and this is a part of everyday routines. Don't forget to make a conscious effort and think about your daily habits regularly. It's an ongoing process.

How Long Does It Really Take for a Habit to Form?

You may have already heard multiple varying answers to this very question. The research from a 2009 study by researchers at University College London reports that it takes, on average, sixty-six days to change a newly developed behavior into a habit. Some more simple tasks, like eating breakfast every day, can become a habit more quickly and more complex or time-consuming behaviors, like cooking dinner four nights a week, can take a little longer. All in all, between three to eight weeks is a good average to keep in mind.

The key to developing and following through with creating a habit is to be very dedicated in those early stages—and then stick with it, each and every day, for at least three weeks. By sticking with something for that long, you give yourself a better chance at having that new habit stay with you, embedded into your routine. Eventually it becomes a natural part of your everyday life.

Here are a few tips:

- Don't bite off more than you can chew! Not in the literal sense (although that certainly can help), but as related to your weekly tasks or goals. You don't need to make too many changes at once, so instead focus on easy tasks at first. Then as those become habits, pick more difficult tasks to focus on.
- Give yourself the right tools you need to make those new changes stick. If you are making exercise a new habit, make sure you have some equipment, even homemade equipment (until you get real weights, soup cans can work), access to a gym, or even a mapped-out route for walking in your neighborhood.
- Get into a routine. Make sure that new behavior is practiced at the same time daily, such as exercising right after work or picking the same time each day to sit down to a family dinner.
- Create a checklist to help you track your accomplishment of those tasks each day.
- Reward yourself appropriately—maybe a manicure, new book, or even a new shirt—once a week for sticking with your new habits. Make sure not to use food as a reward.
- Remember, this is not a race and everyone can be a winner, so if you fall off the wagon, get right back on it tomorrow.

Try thinking of habits as pathways that develop over time, not something that happens overnight. For example, riding your bike down a dirt path that you have never been down before will leave only a small mark in the dirt you can barely even notice. Now, if you ride down that same path every day, you will make a groove in the path that appears to have always been there. The same can be said for neurons. As you develop new habits, you are laying down tracks of neurons on top of each other, strengthening those pathways until your new habit is so entrenched in your daily routine that it becomes second nature to complete. This won't happen overnight and it will take a little time, but give it a try and soon you will see how easy it is to develop healthy habits to allow you to be successful at losing weight. Plus, you won't even believe how effortless those tasks become!

Mom Gave Good Advice: Sit Up Straight

It's amazing, and maybe even hard to believe, but did you know that your brain requires nearly thirty times more blood to flow through it than the other body organs? It's true, so it should be no surprise that anything you do to prevent that blood flow will inhibit the true potential of your brain. Slouching your back will squeeze two arteries that have the task of carrying blood coming from your heart, heading up your spinal column, and taking it all the way to your brain. The act of slumping in your chair, which many of us do each day at work, cuts off the blood supply, and in turn can quickly result in murky thinking and absent-mindedness.

USE BOREDOM TO YOUR ADVANTAGE

Boredom happens when you have reached a limit with what you have learned or can learn when it comes to a skill or topic. Even if you really enjoyed that task or activity at the start, eventually your brain develops the skill needed to perform that required task or action, even to the point where you may (metaphorically of course) say you could do that task "in your sleep." Your brain just doesn't get pleasure from doing the same task over and over again. Without a challenge or stimulation, your brain gets stuck in a rut. While this is not quite the same as forming habits, boredom can quickly turn *into* a habit if you let it!

In addition, boredom can be a vicious cycle and wind up leading to more boredom. If you really want to keep your neurons firing off in top shape, then you need to find something to do that really challenges you. When it comes to diet and exercise, this may include changing up your exercise program or learning to make new healthy recipes in the kitchen. Even meal times and exercise routines can get boring. Anything new you can do will be advantageous. Novelty increases the rewarding feeling that you get when dopamine neurons fire in the brain, which will motivate you to do those new behaviors.

If you think you're stuck in a rut, don't sit idly by and see if it will pass. Boredom is a sure sign that your brain needs new or additional stimulation. Be on the lookout for things that you can do to challenge yourself, like:

1. Strive to be the best at everything you do, even if the task seems small. Commit yourself to putting in a full effort each time, which will push you to new levels.
2. Identify gaps in your abilities (maybe cooking skills or exercise abilities) and fill them up.
3. Continually step it up, challenging your skills and capabilities each day.

Don't let boredom keep you down. When you notice yourself getting into a rut, make sure to challenge yourself. Your weight may depend on it!

MENTAL EXERCISE

All sorts of professional athletes, from football players to gymnasts, routinely run through a focused mental rehearsal before taking part in any competitions. One of the first well-known competitive athletes to openly use this technique was none other than the great boxer Muhammad Ali. He had created for himself a unique way to embrace the power of his mind and use this to his advantage before entering the ring. Just before heading out, Ali used various self-motivational techniques like affirmation, visualization, mental rehearsal, and self-confirmation, including his most famous assertion, "I am the greatest." All of these techniques worked to get him pumped up, with his mind in the game and his eye on the prize.

Can Mental Rehearsal Really Give Healthy Results?

In a recent study conducted at McGill University, Knäuper and team looked at first-year college students and wanted to see what positive influences coming from brain techniques could be used to increase the fruit intake in those who currently had low intake. The control group only used messages of intent each day to help them form their health habit (just repeating their goal). The other groups were given various techniques, including implementation intention (saying their goal and also writing a specific plan), mental imagery (saying their goal but then also imagining themselves doing the behavior), and the final group was asked to do both the mental imagery combined with implementation intention. So, what did they find happened to fruit intake in these college students? Mental imagery (mental rehearsal) did in fact increase fruit intake in those students, and did so even more when paired with implementation intention. Watching yourself do the healthy behavior will help you to better achieve those healthy goals.

So, did this work for Muhammad Ali? You bet it did! He was a top fighter, and focused on exactly what he wanted to gain in life. He used these phrases and sayings not only to pump himself up, but to get the press pumped up too. Most important, he used these to get into the mind of his opponents and intimidate them. Sure, it made a great show and was good for drumming up entertainment, but Ali was moreover creating for himself a very clear mental image of what he wanted to achieve.

The first identification of the brain's ability to employ "dual coding" in the processing of verbal and nonverbal information at the same time was noted by psychologist Allan Paivio, professor emeritus of the University of Western Ontario. He discovered that the mental practice one does for a sport worked just the same as the physical practice when it came to things like timing and patterns. Athletes regularly use this as an accepted training model to help them to learn or improve their skills. Like Ali, you can mentally prepare by using the following techniques!

Visualization Is Not Quite the Same Process

While mental rehearsal many times is assumed to be the same as visualization, these are actually different. With visualization you can be seen as more separated from the act, almost as if you are watching yourself from the outside. Mental rehearsal takes it a step further—in order to work, you need to create very strong images in your mind of actually being there and being present in the actual event or challenge. While eating habits aren't treated the same as competitive sports (well, alright, there is one exception to that one!), learning this training technique can have you in tiptop shape to properly enter the "ring" at meal time.

As always, science is involved in figuring out exactly what is going on, and in this case, researchers determined that the brain can tell the difference between a thought and an action. Researchers looked at a group of skiers and hooked them up to electromyography (EMG) equipment, which measures the electrical impulses your motor neurons send out to specific muscles needed for that activity. The researchers made note of the neural activity experienced by the skiers when they actually were skiing down a hill, but then they also looked at this as they mentally rehearsed the same act. The researchers found that the skiers' brains responded the exact same way whether the skiers were just thinking of the action or if they were really doing it. Even just the thought of the action resulted in the identical mental directions sent from their brain to their body as when they were physically doing the action.

Similarly, research that used an electroencephalogram (EEG), a tool that measures electrical activity within the brain, has produced comparable results. The electrical activity created by the brain is the same whether you are just thinking about doing that action or if you are really, physically doing it. Using this research as a foundation, scientists have theorized that mental rehearsal will create the actual neural pathways you will need to accomplish the real thing. Mental rehearsal can train the brain to make those actions occur with greater ease when it comes time to actually partake in that action. This means there is hope for you yet when it comes to tough food-related decisions, and even getting your physical activity routines up to par. It all comes down to how you use your brain.

You may not be at the same competitive level as an athlete, but the same training skills are still relevant. Just like an athlete has repetitive actions to take in training and performance, you have the same since you have to eat (and are tempted with food choices) each and every day. During an athletic performance, the athlete's brain will release neurotransmitters that signal to the muscles of a specific pathway, and these are stimulated. Those chemicals produced will remain for a short time, so any future stimulation occurring along that very same pathway will benefit as there is some lasting effects from those earlier connections. This repeated practice lays the electrical foundation, and since the brain can't tell the difference between really doing or just thinking it, mental rehearsal can accomplish the same thing and will lay that electrical foundation, just as actual physical practice would. So, when it's time to actually do the action, you have gotten yourself at the top of your game and your body is ready to go, just like you practiced!

Can I Exercise Without Even Moving?

It seems you can. An exercise psychologist at the Cleveland Clinic Foundation, Guang Yue, looked at nonathletic people who made it a habit to hit the gym regularly versus nonathletic people who used the mental rehearsal technique to visualize workouts. The result was that people who frequented the gym increased muscle strength by 30 percent, but people who only worked out in their minds also increased their muscle power—and by nearly half as much as those actually doing the workout physically. Study participants aged twenty- to thirty-five years old simply thought about flexing one of their biceps, doing this as hard as they could, for five times each week. Once it was confirmed they weren't also doing any physical exercise, the researchers noted a very surprising 13.5 percent increase in both muscle size and strength. Even more impressive, this only took a few weeks and the effects lasted three months from the time the visualization exercise took place. You still have to go to the gym to help lose weight, but in your free time you can work out those muscles on your own and be better ready to work out hard when you get to the gym.

For the most effective results, your mental rehearsal is best done during a meditative state, where you have reached top levels of concentration and awareness. When you conjure up thoughts of the future event, design the mental picture to include you right in the middle of all your glory (success in your intended action). Make sure to bring all five senses in as you visualize each part of the task that you will have to complete, down to the very last detail. At the center of your mental picture should be that special moment when you have succeeded in reaching your goal, incorporating how good it feels to have come out on top, and even imagine that your biggest supporters are there cheering you on. It's imperative to really feel the experience just as if it were really happening to you at that exact instant.

TIME TO BEEF UP YOUR FOCUS AND MEMORY SKILLS

The brain has a lot to do each day, and receives a lot of information. According to scientists, we will only remember one out of every 100 pieces of information we receive. Your brain has a hard-working filter that sifts through the information in your working- and short-term memories, tossing out those messages that it doesn't deem vital. Unfortunately, letting your brain take all the action in this process can be chancy because your brain will base this determination on what it has previously been instructed to focus on. So, unless you actively work to reprogram your brain and have it give attention to incoming new bits of information, it isn't going to know what information you truly need saved for later or what you need to have connected with information stored previously.

Alternating Streams

As you learned earlier in this chapter, while it may seem like your brain can focus intently on multiple things at once, the truth is that this just isn't possible. This is why it is so important to focus on each task individually and not do more than one thing at a time. This also applies to eating and grocery shopping, both of which really require your undivided attention. Not giving yourself the proper focus you need to complete all of the tasks that impact your own health will make it that much harder for you to lose the weight and keep it off in the long run.

Snap a Mental Photograph

In order to really remember something, you will want to create an extensive mental picture. Pay attention to all the finer details, and rehearse what you've learned in order to strengthen that memory. Step back in time, to when you were in school, and think about when you were memorizing facts. It's the repetition and the need to remember the information that became a regular part of your day in school. Use those same techniques (seeing, hearing, writing down, and repeating) to boost your memory skills. Having good memory skills helps you along the way by making sure you're better able to remember and utilize all the healthy changes you wish to implement in your everyday life.

The Learning Process

There are three distinct stages when it comes to developing the ability to perform a specific task: learning, retaining, and transferring.

- **Learning:** This happens when you can repeat a new behavior, practically the same, shortly after you were just taught it. For example, you are taught that 1 + 1 = 2, and then you are asked to tell the teacher what 1 + 1 equals. Well, there you have it! You have just learned something, however, this doesn't mean the information is useful unless you are able to remember it and then apply it in other circumstances.
- **Retaining:** This is when you are capable of repeating a newly learned behavior or can utilize the learned information for different circumstances. So, for example, you have retained your addition skills for 1 + 1 when you are asked the question a few days later, doing something completely different, and you're able to give the correct answer.
- **Transferring:** This is when you are able to link new information with old information or with your future learning, and it

happens when you recognize a pattern that matches what you have learned already. So, a few weeks later, you are somewhere else, doing some other activity, and you decide you want one banana and then someone else says they want one too. You think about this and realize that you will need to grab two bananas from the kitchen.

It's clear that these are all different—which is why, for example, you are able to learn to drive a car in good weather, but may have a harder time when it is snowing. It's also why you have an easier time listing out math facts you learned back in middle school, but you can't always easily convert measurements in the kitchen.

Your brain is more efficient when you have mastered the prior step in the learning process before stepping up to the next level, or to starting on something new.

AND SPEAKING OF STARTING SOMETHING NEW . . .

It's finally time to learn the skillful craft of mindfulness and mindfulness meditation, which are two practices that are powerful agents of change in helping you to get thin by improving your brain's abilities. So go ahead and mindfully turn the page!

CHAPTER 8

MEDITATE TO GET THIN

Principle: Focusing your thoughts to regulate your emotions using age-old meditation techniques can help you control that pesky overactive amygdala, all the while strengthening your PFC's ability to focus and function at maximum levels.

To get started, let's take a trip back in history. Let's visit a time where things were simpler and obesity wasn't a problem. It wasn't so hard to clear the mind and focus, taking a time out from the world around us. Back in that simpler time period thousands of years ago, Buddhism developed and with Buddhism came one of the most effective techniques used today to help train your brain: mindfulness, the idea of living in the "here and now." Buddha himself detailed the guiding principles of mindfulness and, today, those Tibetan monks who follow the teachings of Buddha practice mindfulness meditation, which leads to great results in their minds and bodies. These very techniques are the focus of research in the field of neuroscience. Based on that research, there is an increasing number of neuroscientists who agree mindfulness meditation could result in positive changes in your brain function helping you to better achieve your goals.

Think of humans as ever-changing, very dynamic beings, just as they are described based on Buddhist principles. Neuroscientists uncovered scientific evidence to support the concept of neuroplasticity, which is the ability of the human brain to keep growing and forming new synapses. Of course this is great news because it was once thought that this ability was impossible in adulthood. Buddhists, and now neuroscientists, both view human beings as ever changing, with the capability to expand and improve upon the way our minds process and think about information, in turn affecting the overall way our brains work. Learning to take advantage of the concept of mindfulness can help you filter out those thoughts that drift into your brain and have absolutely nothing to do with what is currently going on. Instead, you can make sure that your brain is focused on the "here and now," which will improve your ability to make those wise decisions that are so important when it comes to your eating habits and overall health. It will also help you learn to reduce anxiety, another positive factor in managing weight; stress plays a role in the overall health of the physical body, not just with psychological well-being.

With mindfulness you will learn to be more in tune with your body and the connection between your stomach and your brain. This is very important because appetite is only one part of eating or just wanting food and it is entirely possible to eat when you are not hungry. This is the psychological component to why we eat, not the physiological reason for why we eat, which is known as hunger. Learning to let your body cues of hunger guide you in making food choices, and controlling the brain to prevent unwanted cues of appetite when hunger does not exist, will serve you well on your quest to lose weight.

Without a doubt, one of the biggest benefits you get from mindfulness meditation (or really any form of meditation) is that it assists your brain in strengthening neural pathways associated with achieving your goals. Meditating brings you a better awareness of yourself and, of course, your intentions. It works to strengthen the neuronal connections linked to those specific desires. Alright, let's go take a look at the theories and practices behind mindfulness and see how this process works.

WELCOME THIN MINDFULNESS

Mindfulness is the trained ability in which you nurture the awareness of the present, and do so without depending on those typical and routine responses to events that result in the same old reactions time after time. Basically, this helps you "step outside the box" and assess the current situation with a fresh perspective. This means getting connected to the direct experience right then and there, with all of your brain focused, and not using past experiences to bog you down. This kind of reprogramming will help you to learn new ways to react in various situations and promotes a more positive way to handling these situations. In essence, you are learning how you can control your own mind, instead of having your mind control you.

A main principle of mindfulness is to allow your thoughts to come and go. This means letting thoughts flow freely, not allowing your mind to grasp onto any one thought and drag you back into your standard reactive, or possibly obsessive, tendencies. It helps to break that cycle and let you take control, in a calm and collected way. The practice of mindfulness trains your mind to focus your attention in an overall healthy manner. All your senses are in tune with the present.

From the time we are born, our minds learn how to process internal and external events or stimuli as a specific type of response. We often look at situations and determine whether something is either one thing or the opposite. For example: good or bad, right or wrong, fair or unfair. Instead of going into life events or experiencing situations with an open mind, people tend to respond in a habitual, almost predictable way. You may be guilty of noticing this in others, and it is possible that someone has thought that of you as well. This usual way you have of perceiving and responding may make you quick to jump to the same conclusions or actions, especially if a new experience seems like something else you have encountered in the past. In the end, this does not help you reach your goals.

You may notice that how you felt after some event you experienced in the past affects your current thoughts and even how you may react in similar events in the future. For example, if you felt depressed and sought out food after one time where you weighed yourself and noticed that you gained a couple of extra pounds, this can become your usual reaction every time you see the number on the scale go up. Needless to say, it becomes rather easy to head down the same path and keep on making the same poor choices. The effect of this cycle on health-related decisions, particularly those related to food intake and physical activity, can be a hindrance over time and certainly is not going to contribute to your goal of reaching your healthy and comfortable weight. The practice of mindfulness allows you to develop an awareness of your habitual patterns in thinking. Then you are better able to respond in any situation in a way that is more appropriate to what is really happening at that moment, leaving failed attempts at developing long-term healthy eating habits in the past.

Mindfulness can be a very useful instrument in your journey to find your version of thin, and not someone else's impression of what your weight should be at any given time. Remember that mindfulness has to do with you, and you alone, being aware of the situation and staying in control of your mind when making healthy choices. In addition, mindfulness does more than just help you stay open-minded in the present moment; it also helps you find an awareness of your thought patterns, teaching you how to steer yourself away from any that are unproductive or restrictive. This can be achieved with focused breathing and/or meditation, a concentration technique used to bring yourself into awareness of the present moment. It helps you learn to focus your energy on being right there in the present moment, without being a slave to past circumstances.

The aim of mindfulness is not as much about stopping any of your thought processes as it is about being able to bring your awareness to the present moment and focusing on what is happening right at that time. Living mindfully, combined with meditating mindfully, can help you wash away those negative thought patterns simply by making you aware of them. You have the power to make a conscious decision to break former thought patterns that just haven't worked for you in the past. When you find that you are able to make decisions without holding on to previous thoughts about what you believed were good ways to lose weight, you will be more likely to successfully reach your weight goals.

SO WHY SHOULD YOU MEDITATE?

Meditation, particularly mindfulness meditation, will support your pursuit of a healthy weight by keeping you focused on you personally from a mental, physical, and spiritual standpoint, without letting the negative from your life seep in. When it comes to working toward your healthy goal weight, meditation can:

- Improve blood flow to the brain and muscles, aiding in general good health
- Elevate serotonin levels (the feel-good hormone)
- Decrease cortisol levels (the feel-stressed hormone)
- Improve your sense of inner tranquility
- Construct awareness of your food consumption
- Boost positive decision-making
- Create self-confidence in your choices
- Increase insightful thought processing
- Improve attention spans
- Thicken your cerebral cortex (which may offset age-related cognitive problems)

The benefits of meditation on health are numerous, but even just the relaxation effects and stress reduction alone would make meditation a beneficial component to your weight loss plan.

HOW TO MAKE MEDITATION WORK FOR YOU

Certain thought patterns will help meditation and mindfulness work at their best level. Let's start by looking at this list below to see how to start the process of incorporating meditation into your daily routine. These are key elements to helping you get started with the practice of meditation. You may find it difficult at first to focus and concentrate, but if you stick with it, you will see the rewards.

1. Nurture a beginner's mind. This feature of your "here and now" awareness lets you see things with a fresh outlook, just as if you were seeing them for the very first time, with a sense of wonderment and curiosity.
2. Give up judgment. The goal of practicing mindfulness meditation is to stop jumping to conclusions based on past experiences and labeling thoughts, feelings, or sensations as good or bad, right or wrong, fair or unfair. Instead, you want to get a sense of what is really going on in the situation at that present moment and wipe out all desire to pass judgment. Having a nonjudgmental attitude will help with objectively assessing the situation and coming to a new conclusion.
3. Yield to striving. Striving involves leaping off to reach an endpoint, something further down the road. You can't reach those long-term goals if you don't focus on the right steps in the present that will help you right now. You can't skip steps. Mindfulness is all about your presence in the current moment.
4. Maintain composure. This means at all times. You must keep your cool, even if the situation becomes stressful.

5. Learn to just let it be. Instead of being so focused on results, just let things be without scrutinizing them. Remember that each experience should be treated as new, with new steps to get to the result or desired outcome, and release all preconceived ideas of what should be happening.
6. Build self-reliance. This quality helps you see for yourself, using your own life experiences as research to determine what is true or untrue. This ultimately gives you greater confidence in your decision-making abilities, which in turn will keep you on track as you work toward your goals.
7. Experience self-compassion. With this type of awareness, you can find inner peace while learning to love and accept yourself as is without added pressure or critique.

By taking these first steps on your journey into mindfulness you are learning a new way of clearing your mind and creating a calm sense of being. Meditation will help give you the tools you need to make better decisions related to developing healthy habits.

MEDITATION BONUSES

By practicing and employing mindfulness meditation, you will be better able to handle the ups and downs of staying on track for a healthy lifestyle as you work to find new ways daily to break and change patterns related to failed past attempts at getting to that healthy weight, in addition to cultivating more confidence, initiative, and resourcefulness. You'll learn how to:

- Focus your attention to your choices in a specific way.
- Alert and direct your attention on your actions and behaviors.
- Get rid of distractions and focus your thoughts.
- Monitor and then redirect any hindering emotions.

- Discover and use new ideas for a healthy lifestyle.
- Enhance your creativity.
- Create specific goals to meet your needs.
- Stay right on track and follow through.

Practicing mindfulness meditation helps you in creating the specific intention and motivation your mind needs to change the way it perceives, receives, and reacts to various situations. By practicing mindfulness meditation regularly (once or twice daily for the best results) you will experience a sense of calmness in whatever is happening at that time. This occurs simultaneously while training both your mind and your brain to pay attention and be welcoming to all the thoughts that make their way into your mind. Plus, you will have learned how to do this without passing judgment, and instead doing this with acceptance and open arms—or shall we say minds?

WHY WAIT, START TODAY!

Buddhist master Sakyong Mipham Rinpoche teaches that the easiest way to get started practicing mindfulness meditation is to start by meditating twice a day for short periods of time. Don't stress about finding large blocks of time because those short periods of time may consist of just ten or fifteen minutes. Plus, and this is really good news, you can practice mindfulness meditation anywhere that you feel comfortable and can relax—even right in the comfort and privacy of your home. All you need to do is find yourself a space to claim, which will be your quiet spot for those few minutes twice daily. This could be your bedroom, a spare room, or even a spacious, uncluttered closet. Later, and of course with some practice, you will want to aim for more time each session. Here are some basic guidelines for your mindfulness meditation practice.

Step #1: Build a Space for Your Desired Weight

You can't calm and center your mind without privacy, silence, and tranquility. Some people find it helpful to focus on a small talisman, an object they feel brings them good luck or wards off evil, and will place this on the floor in their view. If you have a talisman, feel free to bring this into your mindfulness meditation routine to assist you as you practice these techniques. Perhaps you may want to use whatever symbol of your goal weight speaks to you, such as a picture of you at that weight previously, those jeans you are hoping to fit back into, or even a bowl of fruit as a reminder of good nutrition.

Step #2: Sit Up Straight

The Buddhist belief is that that energy flows through your body best when you position yourself sitting upright with a straight back, not slouched over. Sitting straight will help you feel elongated and will encourage a better flow of oxygen in and out of your body. To get into this position try balancing yourself on a firm pillow for support, facing your hips straightforward and crossing your legs. Should you find sitting on the floor uncomfortable, try using a chair. Sit up straight, placing your feet flat on the floor. Now place your hands, with palms facing upward, on your thighs. It's not necessary to the practice, but some people like to sit in this pose touching their index fingers and thumbs together, so you can decide what feels most comfortable.

Step #3: Occupy Your Body

Once you have mastered the correct posture, it will be easier for you to focus your undivided attention on both your mind and your body. First, before you even start to meditate, you want to visualize a string starting at the base of your spine that then runs up your back, slowly pulling each vertebra up toward the ceiling and into alignment, then coming all the way through the top of your head. Make sure that as you're sitting, your shoulders and hips are both level on the pillow or cushion. Now make sure you feel completely at one with your body. When done correctly, you will have a relaxed feeling in the awake state; you will not feel drowsy.

Step #4: Reduce Distractions

Some people like to listen to music softly playing in the background as they meditate. If you wish to do this, pick something soothing and relaxing to allow for easy concentration. As your skills develop, you may consider experimenting with guided meditations, which are meditations led by an audio recording. To develop a strict mindfulness practice, leave your eyes open, but keep your gaze a little out of focus and your eyes looking slightly downward, keeping your focus to just about a couple of inches just past your nose. This will help you as you work to control your thoughts and get rid of distractions. Should you find it difficult to focus, consider placing a small object in front of you, on the ground, and use this to refocus your mind anytime it strays.

Step #5: Breathe In the Healthy, Breathe Out the Unhealthy

Learning to control your breathing is a great way to slow down your body and mind. Begin by focusing on each breath. Notice each breath as it flows in and then out of your body. You will want to develop an awareness of your breathing pattern. With your normal breathing, consciously utilize the motion of those breaths to place your body and mind into a state of relaxation. If you happen to be a shallow breather, and are aware that you rarely breathe using your diaphragm, you will want to take it easy as you practice taking those deeper breaths. To help with this, place one hand over your belly button. You can then feel your breaths, as your belly rises and falls, with every inhalation and exhalation, which will help you learn deep breathing.

Step #6: Keep Your Prize in Sight

You should be wholly focused on being fully present in your body and aware of what is going on within your body and mind during mindfulness meditation. When outside thoughts and feelings start to enter your mind, which is only natural, especially when you are just starting out, take notice of where these thoughts have taken you, label them ("distraction," "fear," "something to consider later"), and then rein your mind in, bringing it back to your meditation. Focusing on your breath is a good way to train yourself to come back to the meditation and away from the distracting thought.

Remember that, during meditation, you are teaching your mind a new way to slow down its otherwise busy and quick pace. You are reprogramming the way you perceive and then process information. Basically, you are effectively training your mind to get rid of outside, unnecessary distractions and instead focus 100 percent on one thought at a time.

Step #7: Cool Down

Once you have finished your meditation, you will want to slowly draw your awareness back to your physical setting. Take a few deep, cleansing breaths as a way to tell your body and mind that it is time to move from a focused state of being back into your normal surroundings.

A Meditating Brain Creates a Mindful Brain

Remarkable things are taking place in your brain every time you practice mindful meditation, including:

- When you label your emotions inward with key words, you activate your left PFC, in turn reducing anxiety. Now, on the other hand, if you focus that attention outwardly, labeling those emotions is more likely to activate your right PFC.

- Focusing your concentration reworks the link connecting your thinking brain with the emotional side. As a result, you are strengthening those neuronal pathways directly involved with the higher-level thought process and you are given control of your brain's emotional centers, allowing for a more voluntary identification and control of the emotions you possess.
- Being entirely aware of your surroundings will activate the cortical networks close to your cingulate cortex (the area that increases self-awareness and empathy), the insula (the area focused on internal body states), and the somatosensory cortex (the area designed to sense your body in space), drawing the focus back to you and how you feel in relation to the world around you.
- Allowing yourself to take part in self-observation will activate the medial PFC, which is your center of metacognition and self-relevance, where you have thoughts about thinking or may evaluate your own reasoning.

Without a doubt, all of these benefits to your brain from meditation will nourish you well in your quest to be thin—or, more appropriately, to reach your healthy weight since this will be different for each person.

GET SURFING ON THOSE THETA WAVES

The more your brain systems fire together and in harmony the better your mental health will fare. Mindfulness meditation practiced regularly will increase the activity in your left frontal lobe, while at the same time lowering emotional reactions. Not to mention it will help you become more self-aware, engage in positive thinking, and help you be both sympathetic and empathetic. Mindfulness meditation also gets those ever-so-elusive theta waves (those related to wakeful rest) going, and tunes them along with alpha and gamma waves, in turn producing that elusive feeling of "bliss" so often described by those who regularly meditate.

INCORPORATING MINDFULNESS MEDITATION INTO YOUR LIFE

We all know the saying "practice makes perfect," so it should be no surprise that the more you practice mindfulness meditation, the easier the process will become. You will find the process both soothing and revitalizing, like a small vacation for your mind. Soon you may even find yourself harnessing the energy attained in meditation to help you live fully in the present, remaining conscious of everything in your daily life, which means healthy living in all aspects—staying on track to achieve your weight loss goals.

Looking for Another Option? Try Insight Meditation

Insight meditation is another practice that will help you focus your mind. It starts by first teaching you to be mindful of your inner sanctuary, and then to magnify your awareness to your outside surroundings, including sounds, smells, and so on. When you are outwardly directed with your focus you learn to simply encounter the world as is, without trying to analyze and interpret it, therefore keeping your inner environment unchanging. Massachusetts General Hospital researchers have found an indication that insight meditation will increase the thickness of the gray matter surrounding the right PFC and the right insula (the part of the brain dedicated to your internal state). Practitioners of insight meditation have reported prolonged attention, continuous focus, and an ability to think about something before reacting in new and potentially stressful situations. This can be beneficial to you as you work toward developing new responses to situations involving food choices and healthy lifestyle decision-making.

Once you have developed your mindfulness meditation skills, all you need to do is take a time-out during your day to drop into that relaxed state. It's as easy as taking a quick break, a meaningful time-out in your busy day, to breathe deeply—in and out—and focus yourself, however brief that may be, on being fully present right then, in that moment only. Practicing regularly when you have the time and the urge to clear your mind will assist you in building a mindfulness muscle to help you stay entirely focused on your intentions and your actions as you make changes in your life toward positive health outcomes, both looking and feeling your best.

INTEGRATING MINDFULNESS INTO YOUR LIFE

The next step after mastering mindfulness meditation is putting it into practice and living mindfully. This is no easy task to master, but you will be well on your way, empowered with the tools you need for success. It's way too easy to stay in your comfort zone, letting your daily routines and habits chip away at your best intentions. As you may know all too well, this can leave you feeling powerless and out of touch with whatever is happening around you . . . or even internally. Living mindfully includes paying attention to what is taking place within your body and your external surroundings in that present moment—without making judgments. It means you stay aware of what is happening around you instead of just jumping to your usual thought patterns and actions—or, better yet, your reactions.

Your brain was constructed to categorize and analyze *everything* that your senses pick up, including tastes and smells, which are so important when it comes to your body's response to foods. So, unless you are willfully steering your brain it can in fact turn around, taking you off course while you get lost in your habitual thoughts. Working on getting your brain focused on reality, what's happening right then and there, via mindfulness meditation and getting those neuronal paths opened up, will provide a direct route to your success.

Living Mindfully Practice #1: Mini-Meditation

A few times daily take a moment to pause, shut your eyes, and focus your breathing until your mind settles down. As thoughts flow into your brain, allow them to drift away by gently bringing your mind back to your breathing, inhaling and exhaling, forcing out whatever is going on in your outside surroundings. Stay in the "mini-meditation" for around five minutes, and down the road you can build this up to fifteen-minute sessions. With practice, and practice does make the difference, you can learn to silence any inner-mind conversations that have been distracting you. This is a great way to bring back your focus when you find that your mind has been roaming.

Living Mindfully Practice #2: Be Completely Present

Another way to practice mindfulness is by being completely aware of, and taking a conscious role in, what you select to do in every waking moment. For example, if you are prepping vegetables for your salad, bring your entire attention to that task, focusing on the activity at hand. Put all external and internal conversations on hold and focus your attention on the sharpness of the knife as the blade slices through those vegetables, with the crunch of your knife as it moves through the fibrous parts of food, touching down with the cutting board, and the connection you make as you feel the texture and taste the salad as a forkful enters your mouth and you start to chew.

You will quickly discover that living mindfully can be very efficient at drowning out the distractions of your busy life, silencing a chattering mind and training your brain to focus instead on enjoying the moment you are in. This in turn will help you form a healthy relationship with the foods you are consuming.

As you practice these simple techniques more and more, and reinforce them by meditating mindfully, the more you will train your brain to allow you to accomplish whatever you need it to do. You will find that your training helps you do this efficiently—helps you get to your perfect weight and provides you with good health and happiness both inside and outside. Nothing will please you more than the control and inner peace you will feel over making the right healthy lifestyle choices.

LIVING AND MEDITATING MINDFULLY CAN TAKE YOU TO YOUR IDEAL WEIGHT

When it comes to attaining your ideal weight, teaching your brain to be more perceptive, more zoned in to your daily food choices, and more aware of your habits will really benefit you when it comes to making decisions. This will allow you to evaluate your food choices more rationally and logically, backed by a greater education of the power of eating the right foods. You will be better able to make those decisions about what to eat without letting your emotions take over and choosing those foods for you.

Mindfulness meditation basically rewires your brain to allow you to break free from your normal pattern of reaction to new experiences, which often happens automatically based on your previous encounters and experiences. With meditation, the goal is not to put the brakes on your emotional responses to what's going on in your life, but to help you avoid reacting out of habit, hindering you from moving forward. This could prove a helpful tool in dealing with tough changes to your eating habits and patterns and training yourself to break the cycle of yo-yo dieting. It may also help you manage better when you feel like someone is sabotaging your progress or does not understand your desire to make better food choices daily. You are in control of your food choices, and only you can make those decisions. Mindful meditation can help guide you away from negative thoughts about what you are and are not capable of, leaving you stronger when faced with tough food choices. It serves as a reminder that, when push comes to shove, you control your reactions.

Therefore, by instituting the practice of meditation to your daily routine, you are amplifying your brain's ability to function optimally and expand, both of which are critical in helping you reach your goal weight. So what are you waiting for? Go ahead—grab a comfy pillow, sit right down, and let the breathing begin!

CHAPTER 9

PLAY YOUR WAY TO THIN

Principle: Your brain benefits from periods of stimulation and periods of relaxation—and it enjoys learning new skills.

Partaking in playful activities stimulates those portions of your brain that often go unused, creating new synapses and making sure you don't get stuck in neuronal ruts. Play also offers stress relief (by reducing cortisol), burns calories, and can make you happier, all of which lead you to greater success in getting thin. There is also a link between creativity and play—play can stimulate your creative juices and help you come up with new or better ways to incorporate healthy living into your daily practice.

WHY PLAY IS VERY IMPORTANT

Have you ever noticed that most kids look happy most of the time? There is a reason for this. Have you guessed it yet? It's because they are given the chance, and even encouraged, to play each and every day. Since most adults work, we are not given the same time dedicated to play, which is a shame because play is actually an essential part of brain health throughout your entire life—in fact, it may even be more important as you get older. Play helps foster a healthier brain and promotes great brain function. And it is not only fun, but also a great way to reduce stress and stimulate your mind. So, just how playful are you?

The *How Much Do You Play* Quiz

1. You play hooky from work:

A. once every few weeks.
B. once every few months.
C. one to two times a year.
D. What's hooky?

2. You have sex:

A. three or more times per week.
B. once weekly.
C. once monthly.
D. can't remember.

3. To you, a mental challenge would be:

A. learning a new language.
B. completing the *New York Times* Crossword puzzle.
C. beating the final level of your favorite video game.
D. watching a trivia TV show.

4. You'd be most likely to splurge on:

A. a weekend getaway trip.
B. a relaxing day at the spa.
C. a brand new outfit for work.
D. new shoes.

5. You consider a physical challenge for yourself to be:

A. training for a half marathon.
B. joining a noncompetitive team sport with friends.
C. going to the gym once or twice weekly.
D. walking to the kitchen.

6. **You take vacations:**

   A. Isn't every weekend is a vacation?

   B. twice yearly.

   C. annually.

   D. I can't remember the last time I took a vacation.

7. **You really enjoy a good game of:**

   A. geocaching.

   B. Words with Friends.

   C. Go Fish.

   D. I haven't played a game in ages.

8. **When I want to learn something new, I usually:**

   A. revel in my progress, even giving myself small rewards.

   B. create a list of goals and cross them off as I accomplish them.

   C. quit before completely learning it.

   D. move on to something else, and the feeling will eventually pass.

Answer Key

If you checked mostly As, you have already done a good job making play a vital component in your life, but there are still benefits to letting yourself to play harder.

If you checked mostly Bs, you indulge in play every once in a while, but you still need to carve out more time out for fun, allowing your brain the break it needs for a little relaxation and play.

If you checked mostly Cs, you have lost track of your playful side and can't remember how good it feels to play. You've fallen victim to a busy life and are probably a little stressed out. It's time to get up and get out and play. Go have some fun. Your brain will thank you for it!

If you checked mostly Ds, your life is missing a key component to happiness and a healthy brain. All work and no play is dragging you down and really putting a damper on your life. All that stress may be preventing you from losing weight—even worse, it could be helping you put it on!

BRAIN PLAY

As you learned right at the start of this book, the more positive energy you have, the more success you will have managing your weight. Playing not only stimulates pleasure centers in your brain, but also rejuvenates your brain and allows you to enter a more relaxed state. Basically, engaging in playful activities stimulates your brain to think that things are fun or that you are having fun in whatever you are doing. To capitalize on this feeling and reinforce those good feelings, your brain sends out the neurotransmitter dopamine, which is typically thought of as the "pleasure" chemical. In addition, your brain also sends out chemicals that make you feel good, such as oxytocin, vasopressin, and endorphins, which promote a positive and happy outlook. Avoiding negative thinking and depression will make it easier to make smart decisions that impact your daily choices about food and physical activity.

Do you want to play your way to a thin body? Then, let's get started.

NOVELTY IS THE WAY TO GO

By now you should know that presenting your brain with fresh experiences will help it form new neuronal pathways. The more often you do an activity, the more synapses are fired in your brain, the more new synapses will be created. Novelty is wonderful because it stimulates those dormant synapses that have become inactive or it will cause the creation of new synapses altogether. Just remember that your brain will adapt and expand to understand and process the information that *you* consider valuable.

Play to Get Thin

You may think that kids get to have all the fun, but that's not true. Maybe when you were a kid your parents signed you up for football or maybe soccer. There is no reason why getting older means you can't have fun with a team sport. In fact, many cities now have sports leagues aimed at adults. Not only will this kind of play engage your mind, but it will also get your heart pumping and burn calories at the same time, meaning you get double the benefit. The Centers for Disease Control and Prevention (CDC) data on physical activity in 2009 shows that only 47 percent of adults over the age of eighteen are meeting the guidelines for aerobic physical activity, which means many people are still not getting in enough exercise. Don't think of exercise as only going for a run or getting on the treadmill. Think like a kid and get out there and play a sport!

One reason why play is important in your life is because it opens you up to new experiences and forces your brain out of any rut it gets stuck in. One approach to play is trying something different, something you have not done before. It really doesn't matter *what* you do, just as long as this is something that will present a mental challenge. Finding something that you think is fascinating or exciting will strengthen your desire to stick with it. Of course, you will never know how much you enjoy something until you try it, so don't pass over things you think you may not like until you've at least tried it once. This book will start you off on the right path by sharing general activities known stimulate the brain. Once you are in the swing of things, though, you will want to create your own list of things that you find fun and will engage your brain to help you lose weight.

Recently, San Francisco State University researchers found that people who master a skill experience a greater sense of happiness, no matter what level of difficulty it took to become proficient in that skill. As long as you enjoy the activity, you will be happier—but of course it is suggested to try out activities that also work to stimulate your brain. Let's get you started with just a few ideas:

- **Learn a musical skill.** Learning to read music and play an instrument consistently proves to be a powerful method to shape your brain that few other activities have the ability to do. If you've already mastered music, try something else like painting or golf. Just as long as you challenge your mind and your coordination by learning something new, you will have the benefit of growing from the experience, and will increase your happiness.
- **Start an active living blog.** You don't want to increase your time spent in front of a computer, but the idea of keeping a public, online blog about how you are staying active can help you learn something new. Not to mention this will boost your creativity in finding new ways to stay active when you aren't blogging about it.
- **Learn about photography.** In this age of digital cameras it is easy to take photos, but there is also a lot that goes into the art of photography. Learning how to perfect your photography skills will teach you something new and can keep you active as you search for new material to focus your lens on.
- **Learn how to play complex card games.** This is an exceptional way to strengthen your mind by improving your math skills and challenging your working memory. This will also help you develop better skills at reading people. While online games are just as good for the mind, if you are managing your weight it is best to limit time spent in front of the computer. Playing with a group of people in person is a better way to make sure you get your body moving while working out your mind.

No matter what you decide to pick up as a new hobby, make sure it is something that holds your attention and that you find fun. After all, it's hard to stick with something that you don't enjoy. Finding something to stimulate your brain in new ways will keep your brain active and prevent it—and you—from falling into a rut.

The Life Expectancy of Neurons

Your neurons start forming while you are in your mother's womb, and can live well up to 100 years, or even longer! The original thought was that these couldn't be replaced when they died, but new evidence shows that neurons can be generated in some of the brain regions, even if you are older. This is why it is important to keep providing stimulation to your brain. Not only will this improve the life expectancy of your existing neurons, but it will also help to generate new ones in your hippocampus, the learning and memory center. And while your body can take care of fixing up its own cells, it's your job to provide the stimulation necessary to keep your brain cells ticking.

PLAY FOR FUN AND FAT LOSS

While negative thinking can bring your spirits down and lead to a depressed brain, positive thinking and activities that bring joy will do just the opposite. Not only will this benefit your brain, but it will benefit your body, too. Playing is all about enjoying yourself, having fun, and boosting good spirits and a positive outlook on life. This may seem like a difficult undertaking, especially if you spend a lot of time at work or taking care of the more serious matters in your life, but keep reading to see just how easy it can be to incorporate more play into your life.

Pleasure Versus Enjoyment

Do you know the difference between something pleasurable and something enjoyable? Take a moment to think about this. Pleasure is the feeling you get when you have satisfied a physical need such as hunger, thirst, sexual desire, or bodily comfort. Enjoyment is a little different. This is something that you feel when you experience something outside of what you thought were your limits, both physically and mentally. You get enjoyment from:

- Accomplishing a feat that pushed past your known limits.
- Surpassing the expectations set by yourself and others.
- Partaking in stimulating conversations.

Pleasure does serve a purpose, but it is enjoyment that will help you feel good about yourself and reach your weight and healthy lifestyle goals in the long run.

Don't Cloud Your Mind

Chronic stress leads to many health problems, takes the fun out of the day, and even impacts how you think. Studies continue to show those health risks from stress, but what you may not know is that chronic stress also wreaks havoc on your brain—it clouds your mind and shrinks the part of your brain attached to memory and learning. Even worse, it impacts the function of your neurotransmitters—including those that make you feel happy—and releases toxins into your brain. Stress is just no good! So sit back, relax, and do your mind and body a favor by destressing. You shouldn't let life be all work and no play . . . get out there and have some fun!

Ready, Set, Reward!

If you often find yourself in a stressed-out state, making plans for something you find fun is essential to getting your stress under control and helping you manage your weight. Just the act of enjoying something can offer some benefits, including stimulating the positive thinking areas of your brain. Any time you switch it up and stray from your routine, you will develop new thought patterns and see things in a new light.

To start, grab a piece of paper and a pencil and first jot down a list of five activities that bring you pleasure and then jot down five activities that bring you enjoyment. Moving forward, use these as a guide and see those new thought patterns develop.

Things that may bring you pleasure:

- Cooking dinner using a new recipe
- Trying out a new cuisine
- Going out on a date
- Getting a great deal on a piece of furniture
- Test-driving a fast car

Things that may bring you enjoyment:

- Building a model plane
- Planning a trip across Europe
- Learning a new language
- Painting a mural
- Learning to play tennis

Most important, you want to make sure that these are your own lists. Spend some time thinking about what brings you pleasure and enjoyment. Let your brain lead the way. You may even surprise yourself with the creative ideas you come up with. Once you have your list, go ahead and challenge yourself each month to come up with novel ideas and implement a few them. While they may not all pan out, the entire process from start to finish is a good exercise to get your brain stimulated. Make sure to fully take the time to live in the moment and enjoy the experience. Revel in your accomplishments. This way, on those days when you're feeling a little down or bored, you can relive those memories, allowing your brain to re-experience that same enjoyment.

Anticipation Stimulation

There is something to be said for anticipation. Sometimes this feeling is even better than the real thing. *Anticipating* rewards coming in the future stimulates the pleasure centers in your brain's limbic system, just in the same way *experiencing* the actual event will. Ever get butterflies in your stomach and a giddy feeling just before going on a date? This happens because your brain acknowledges everything that leads up to the event. All you have to do is think of something that will give you those same butterflies and giddy feeling, which produce that same anticipation. Nothing is out of bounds here so, even if it seems impossible, picture every single detail of what you want to happen. Don't forget that intensely picturing something has the power to trick your brain into making it think that that action is really happening, just as if you were really there.

FIND YOURSELF A HOBBY!

It's alright if you already have a regular hobby. This means you already know the pleasure you can get from participating in something just for the fun of it. But, if you don't have already have a hobby, you will want to find one. This is important because hobbies give you the chance to stimulate parts of yourself that are otherwise not stimulated in your everyday life. Some hobbies may go back to your childhood. Perhaps you had a hobby that really brought you pleasure, and therefore you make sure to still do it. Or maybe you would like to keep doing it if you just had the spare time.

It's important to make finding time for a hobby—whether it's collecting action figurines, knitting, or building furniture—a priority. Working hard is important, but in order to be successful you need a little quality time for yourself. After all, without a little playtime, you can't keep your brain in tip-top shape! In the end, it really doesn't matter what you pick for your hobby. It only matters that you *love* what you're doing.

Hobbies give you a chance to escape from work or other responsibilities and unwind a little, pushing stress to the backburner. It is also always a nice feeling of accomplishment when you produce something tangible, such as a piece of art, a scarf, or beautiful black-and-white photos, all of which are things you can show off to family and friends later on. Being happy in what you are doing and getting to show something off that you find to be fun also help boost concentration, which in turn increases the chemicals that energize your brain.

In addition, hobbies also benefit you by:

- Stimulating new ideas. Making new neural connections that can then be carried over into your work and personal life.
- Developing your sense of commitment, which then results in a greater level of neuronal engagement and helps you feel as if you have accomplished something.
- Activating more areas in your brain, including some that you may never have stimulated before.
- Creating a new and improved version of *you*, boosting your self-esteem.

Ideally, the hobby you choose should engage your brain, provoke your inner passion, and expand your social connections, all the while giving you a feeling of fulfillment and achievement. Don't forget to start off your hobby by engaging your intellectual side. This can be done with a little research before jumping right in, and also include a social aspect such as attending dance lessons, art classes, or gardening clubs.

This may even give you the push you needed to make other changes in your life that may be making you unhappy. It's not uncommon for people to find that the things they thought would make them happy actually don't, and finding hobbies can spark a new career path.

A Fun Way to Work Out

Don't let your body woes stand in the way of having fun. You might think sex is just a way to make your body feel good, but there is more to it than that. Not only is it good for the brain, but also you get to burn some calories in the process. Having sex really does produce a sense of euphoria, both physically and emotionally. Having sex releases dopamine and endorphins, neurotransmitters that provide you with a sense of pleasure and make you feel good all over. Having an orgasm provides you with a nice, healthy, and naturally occurring dose of dopamine, as well as the bonding neurotransmitter oxytocin. Dutch researchers scanned the brains of volunteers while they were experiencing orgasm. These scans showed that the volunteers were experiencing a rush similar to what people feel when they use heroin. What a great way to enjoy your time, reduce stress, burn some calories, and ultimately get you closer to your healthy weight!

SOCIALIZE WITH YOUR COLLEAGUES

Humans aren't created to be solitary beings. We are designed to want to have those connections with others. When you are with people you value and respect, your brain releases endorphins, giving you a pleasant feeling. Studies have demonstrated that when you make connections with other people who make you feel supported and nurtured, these connections help to improve your health and keep you happy. How? Well, letting your social brain do its thing will stimulate your pleasure-seeking limbic system, all the while putting a muzzle on your ever-fearful amygdala. Basically, simply hanging around and engaging in social activity with people you admire, mentors, and colleagues will help you reduce anxiety and boost your success.

LAUGH YOURSELF THIN

"A good time to laugh is any time you can." Journalist Linda Ellerbee couldn't have been more right. Laughing seems to incite a response in three areas of your brain. You have a response from your PFC, which helps you get the meaning of the joke; the supplementary motor cortex sends the message to your facial muscles allowing them move; and areas of your limbic system promote that giddy feeling. What makes each individual laugh will be different, and the underlying cause really is a mystery, but what is known is that laughing has positive rewards—and that you can and should do it whenever you see fit.

Say Cheese!

Research shows that even just smiling can brighten your mood. Studies have demonstrated that babies smile around 400 times a day and toddlers smile about 300 times a day. What about adults? Well, that's a little less . . . on average they smile only fifteen times to twenty daily. So, whenever you're feeling blue, get up and stroll around your office smiling at your colleagues. Before you know it, someone will tell a joke or share a funny story and your mood will be lifted.

Laughter works to lighten the mood and works to get others around to join in and laugh too. In addition, laughter promotes a bevy of health benefits. It reduces stress hormones, particularly cortisol; it works to lower blood pressure; reduces the risk of developing blood clots; aids in a strong immune system; and helps promote the release of endorphins. Really, when it comes down to it, it doesn't matter what makes you laugh or when you do it, because any laughter will help you feel better, no matter how brief it may last.

THE FUN HASN'T ENDED

We hope this chapter gave you some inspiration to find space in your life for having a lot more fun—not only to keep you in a positive mood and reduce stress, but also to provide some much-needed brain stimulation. The next stop on your journey will be a discussion of exercise and why it is important for both your weight and your brain.

CHAPTER 10

EXERCISE YOURSELF THIN

Principle: Your brain relies upon you to do whatever it takes to keep it healthy, which includes keeping your body healthy and the blood circulating.

It isn't news that exercise is an integral part of managing your weight. And you probably know that working out is also good for general health and promoting your overall sense of well-being. But you may not know that physical activity—and more specifically aerobic exercise—helps manage your weight indirectly as well by:

- Stimulating circulation and increasing blood flow around your body, to your extremities, and particularly to your brain.
- Keeping your brain supplied with the energy it needs to help it stay receptive and flexible.
- Increasing healthy growth factors located within your brain's memory center and elsewhere.
- Improving coordination between your muscles, helping your brain think at its maximum potential.
- Increasing your self-esteem, making you feel good and promoting a strong sense of confidence—not just for your body, but in other aspects of your life.

In this chapter you will learn about the benefits of physical activity and how this can impact your efforts at losing weight and being healthy. You may have thought that the benefit of working out was only that you burn calories and this helps you lose weight, but there is a lot more to exercise than just that!

HOP ON THE EXERCISE TRAIN

When you hear the word exercise, it is likely thoughts of a gym pop into your head. The good news is that exercise has moved beyond the gym, and physical activity can really take place anywhere. You no longer need to feel like you have to be in the gym to get in a good workout. There are plenty of other ways to burn off those calories and stimulate your mind that you find more fun and better fit for your lifestyle. Let's take a moment to see how you're doing on the exercise front.

The *What's My Physical Activity Level* Quiz

1. I participate in at least 30 minutes of exercise:

A. five days each week.
B. three days each week.
C. twice monthly.
D. never.

2. My idea of the perfect workout is:

A. running with a good friend, as we train for an upcoming race.
B. playing basketball with my coworkers.
C. taking a walk around my neighborhood.
D. sleeping.

3. When I don't have a lot of time, I:

A. wake up earlier to make sure I fit in my workout.
B. fit in a short, at-home workout with an exercise DVD.
C. put working out on hold until my schedule opens up.
D. don't think twice about cutting exercise out of my plan.

4. I find exercise to be:

- **A.** a lot of fun and enjoyable.
- **B.** essential to my health.
- **C.** something that needs to be done, even though I don't like it.
- **D.** dreadful.

Answer Key

If you picked mostly As and Bs, you have a good level of physical activity already built into your daily routine. This is great! You know the importance of exercise for keeping your body fit, and now you know this is good for your brain too. You may find from time to time that you get bored or reach a plateau in your weight loss, so don't forget to mix it up a little and introduce new components to your already well-designed routines.

Before You Get Started

Not sure how much exercise to aim for? Looking at the National Weight Control Registry, which documents the habits and lifestyle aspects of more than 10,000 people who have lost significant weight and kept it off, 90 percent of individuals reported doing at least 1 hour of exercise per day. According to Healthy People 2020, the U.S. government's 10 year plan for improving its citizens' health, the current aims are: to work to "reduce the proportion of adults who engage in no leisure-time physical activity" and "increase the proportion of adults who engage in aerobic physical activity of at least moderate intensity for at least 150 minutes/week, or 75 minutes/week of vigorous intensity, or an equivalent combination." This is at a minimum, so the best place to aim is 30 to 60 minutes of physical activity 5 days a week. But, there is no need to jump right in and start off above your capabilities. Start slowly and work your way up.

If you picked Cs or Ds, you will want to reconsider your relationship with exercise and physical activity. In order to lose weight, keep it off, and have your brain help you along the way, you need to tone your body and your mind!

Ode to Your Noggin

University of California–Irvine researchers have shown that the changes noted in your brain resulting from exercise happen because exercise stimulates release of proteins that improve brain function called *neural growth factors.* These neural growth factors, which include brain-derived neurotorophic factor (BDNF), can boost synapse number, as well as the number of new neurons via neurogenesis. Exercise will grow new brain cells and is a vital component for helping your brain stay active and flexible, which is especially important as you age.

OH WHAT A (STRESS) RELIEF!

As you know, play is a great way to relieve stress, and exercise is a great way to play. Not only will you get the benefit of feeling better after you work out, but you get the very important benefit of burning stored energy, helping you shed the excess weight and getting you closer to your thin body and healthy weight. Exercise is also very beneficial because getting rid of the stress, coupled with a great sense of success and accomplishment from finishing your workout and meeting your exercise goals, will allow you to make better decisions both for healthy eating choices and for a healthy lifestyle in general.

Defy Aging

One of the most amazing things about exercise is that the effects it has on your brain are endless, and actually become even more beneficial for your brain health as you age. Neuroscientists have demonstrated that in aging populations, typically people sixty-five and older, the participation in moderate exercise enhances seniors' learning and memory. This was shown to improve their insightful brain function and work against age-related, and even disease-related, mental decline. This was also shown to protect against atrophy related to aging in those areas of the brain that are essential to thinking and learning. Not surprisingly, exercise has been cited by several researchers, including University of California–Irvine researchers, as being the number-one influence for helping maintain brain health with age and in the ability to generate new neurons as we get older.

TRIPLE YOUR BENEFITS

You know that exercise helps maintain weight and helps relieve stress, but there is one more benefit to exercise. You have probably guessed by now that exercise also targets those pleasure centers in your brain, particularly if you have an exercise routine or physical activity that you really find to be fun. Plus, it doesn't matter much what activity you do as long as you get your heart pumping (although toning your muscles is beneficial, too). As long as you get up and move often, you can stimulate your brain's ability to function. When it is something that you enjoy, the neural links made between pleasure and exercise will work to reinforce the behavior and you will want to work out even more! Here are some ideas to get you started, so just make sure you pick something that fits your skill level:

- Try yoga
- Sign up for a 5K or 10K race
- Join an adult league sports team, like flag football or soccer
- Try a new aerobics class
- Go hiking
- Take a ballroom dancing class
- Learn how to kick box
- Ride your bike more often
- Swim laps at a local pool
- Learn martial arts

Just remember, what works for your family members and friends may not be the best fit for you. Pick your activities based on your likes and what you enjoy doing. It's not worth investing your time in the activity if you end up feeling like it is a chore.

GETTING TO THIRTY

One of the reasons that physical activity guidelines recommend working out for thirty minutes most days as a minimum is because this helps in the prevention of many chronic diseases. However, to lose weight or maintain a weight loss you'll have the most success aiming for sixty minutes most days, but you may want to start out at thirty minutes, especially if you are currently not getting any time in or are new to working out. In addition, when it comes to brain health, it only takes thirty minutes most days of something as simple as a brisk walk or a yoga video that you can do in your living room. These simple activities, coupled with other kinds of regular exercise weekly, will work to tone your body and your mind. To make getting that thirty minutes in even easier, keep in mind that you don't have to work out for thirty consecutive minutes; you can break this up for a cumulative effect. For example, taking a brisk walk, or whatever activity you enjoy, for just ten minutes three times daily, will provide you with a benefit. When working out to lose weight, you may find it easier (time-wise) to fit in a structured workout of thirty minutes, coupled with three ten-minute walking sessions each day, and maybe in time you will find that you can fit in a full sixty minutes of exercise most days of the week.

When an Apple Is Bad

Maybe you have heard of people described as apples and pears. Being described as an apple means you carry extra fat tissue around the midsection of your body. While this is typically described as more common in men, it does occur in both genders. Not only does the extra bulge around your midsection put you at a higher risk for disease, but it can eventually take on a life of its own. Those abdominal fat cells have the ability to produce their own hormones, which can impact your brain. For example, fat cells produce leptin, the hormone that regulates satiety, or fullness during and between meals. When you are overweight and have too many fat cells, your body overproduces leptin and your brain no longer listens to the signal that you are full, resulting in overeating. These abdominal fat cells can also release cytokines, the very same inflammatory chemicals released by your body in response to an infection or an injury. The excess quantity of cytokines can have a negative impact on your brain, as they have been linked to many brain-related conditions, including depression, decreased long-term memory capabilities, and a reduction in the plasticity of your brain.

Man's Best Weight Loss Tool!

If you don't own a dog, maybe it's time you give it some consideration. A study published by researchers at Michigan State University looked at the exercise habits of 5,900 people. Of those,

2,170 owned dogs and, not surprisingly, about two-thirds of those dog owners regularly walked their pet for at least ten minutes at a time. Out of those dog owners that regularly walked their pets, 60 percent were meeting the federal guidelines for regular, moderate, or vigorous exercise. Just about half of those dog owners were exercising for an average of thirty minutes daily, on at least five days each week. Compared to dog owners, roughly a third of those who were non–dog owners regularly exercised that much.

Researchers also found that the people regularly walking their dogs also spent more time participating in other moderate and vigorous physical activities than those who did not regularly walk dogs. They were more likely to enjoy other forms of physical activity, like sports. On average, they were exercising for around thirty more minutes each week than people without dogs to walk.

More positive effects of having a dog to walk were shown in a study of 41,500 dog-owning California residents. They were found to be around 60 percent more likely to walk leisurely than those residents without a dog to walk. In the end, that added up to dog owners getting an extra nineteen minutes a week of walking. Not a bad benefit to having a dog to walk. There is even more research showing positive results for dog owners. Plus, you aren't just getting exercise (good for the heart!), stimulating your brain, and enjoying the fresh air; you are also burning more calories in the process, helping you to shed the pounds.

In a twelve-week study conducted at the University of Missouri, researchers looked at fifty-four subjects, all older adults in an assisted-living facility. Results indicated that dogs, not humans, make better companions for walking. Some participants picked a human to be their walking companion, but others decided to take a bus each day to a nearby animal shelter, where they were given a dog to take out with them for a walk. While the walking speed may have increased in both groups of people, it only increased 4 percent for those walking with humans. For those walking dogs, walking speed increased by

28 percent. Dr. Johnson, the study's lead author, and coauthor of *Walk a Hound, Lose a Pound*, found that those walking with other people tended to complain more often to each other (specifically about the heat), and often talked each other out of exercising. On the other hand, people walking dogs didn't make those excuses, making them more successful at spending more time walking.

Turn Those Wheels

New research gives another boost to the mounting evidence for exercise and brain health. Using mice, Illinois professor Justin S. Rhodes from the Beckman Institute for Advanced Science and Technology, designed four living situations that looked at mental stimulation and exercise. One group was given a tasty diet with nuts and cheeses, and their rooms were decorated nicely and complemented with toys. The next group had a similar set up, but they also had the addition of a running wheel. The next group was given bland living quarters, complemented by a bland diet, and the final group was also given the same, but with the addition of a running wheel. After observing the mice performing various cognitive tests, it was demonstrated that stimulation, like toys, did not improve brain function. Do you know what did? Hopefully you guessed exercise. Regardless of the way the room looked and the availability of toys, the mice had healthier brains when exercise was involved. Rhodes stated in a recent article, "Only one thing mattered and that's whether they had a running wheel."

Are you convinced yet? If not, consider this interesting finding as well. Not only do pets make loving companions, but they also provide additional health benefits that extend beyond just getting you to exercise more. Dr. Karen Allen looked at forty-eight stockbrokers, all of whom were diagnosed with high blood pressure (a.k.a. hypertension). To give you an idea about blood pressure numbers, normal blood pressure values are less than 120 for the systolic number and less than 80 for the diastolic number. When talking about high blood pressure, stage 1 is classified as 140–159 for systolic values and 90–99 for diastolic. Stage 2 is just a little higher with those cut-off values being 160 or greater for systolic and 100 or greater for diastolic. So knowing what is normal and what is high, let's see how those stockbroker test subjects fared. Those participants who had pets at home were found during stressful situations to have their resting systolic blood pressure increase to only 126. Those without pets were noted to have a greater increase, going all the way up to 148. Not to mention that Dr. Blair Justice from the University of Texas has also found positive results to having a dog. It was noted that just ten minutes of playtime with a dog stimulates your brain to release dopamine and serotonin, two feel good neurotransmitters that can improve your mood and even help you resist food cravings.

But remember that being a dog owner is a lot of work and responsibility. Carefully evaluate if you have the time, money, and space to properly care for a dog before you take this big step and become a dog owner. This does require extensive research and should not be a decision made lightly.

NOT A FAN OF EXERCISE?

If you aren't a big fan of exercising, or any type of physical activity, the perfect solution is to trick your mind! That's right, trick yourself into a newfound love of exercise. Even if you can think of tons of reasons why you hate exercise and would never want to do it, perhaps even remembering failed past attempts, we have the solution for you: reward your brain!

Make It Pleasurable

You might as well rewire your brain to find pleasure in exercise. If you are truly serious about getting rid of the weight and keeping it off, you need to make a lifelong commitment to physical activity—so stop feeling like you're punishing yourself and start having some fun! Let's say that you have a new exercise routine you want to start, and it's something that you've tried and failed at in the past. In order to generate new neuronal pathways to support, not lessen, your will to succeed, you will want to consciously use your mind to link the new activity to something that you consider rewarding. Maybe that new activity would be socializing with your colleagues after playing a round of golf, or perhaps going out for a cup of coffee with your workout buddy after you finish at the gym. Whatever reward you pick, make sure this is something that you really find to be fun. Then just stick with it, doing it each time you exercise.

It is important that you reward yourself either during or right after you participate in whatever activity you choose. This will help your brain link up the new activity with positive feelings, which in turn will reinforce the development of more positive connections within your brain. In no time you will find that your new physical activity is something you actually enjoy, and eventually you won't need to provide that reward to make the activity seem fun.

Shake Those Bad Habits

On the other hand, if you are looking to train your brain to get rid of negative habits, you will want to teach it to deem those habits neutral. Stop linking negative thoughts to rewards or punishments. For example, instead of getting upset because you weren't able to work out one day, don't jump to attach a negative or positive emotion, thought, or action. Instead, neutralize that negative thought. This way you have made sure that your negative thoughts about your habits are stopped. While this isn't going to suddenly make you see these habits as positive ones, this will help you to reduce feelings of stress or anxiety over something you have labeled as negative in your life. Let your brain know that your habit is neither good nor bad. It is just a habit that you have, and you can move forward from there.

Now, if neutralizing doesn't work for you, the next time you skip your workout, force yourself to do something you don't enjoy. Maybe for you that is scrubbing your bathrooms, or cleaning out your closet—but whatever this is for you, it needs to be something you truly dislike. Then you should force yourself to do that activity each time you skip a workout. Sure enough, you will soon find that skipping those workouts just isn't worth the pain of putting yourself through the torturous activity, and in time you will have kicked that bad habit to the curb.

The more power that your mind has over your emotions and thoughts when it comes to the bad habits you want to ditch, the more your brain will work to get rid of those neuronal connections that have been dragging you down that same old road.

EXERCISE GOT YOU TIRED?

No need to worry if all that exercise talk has left you exhausted. In the next chapter you'll learn how sleeping can aid your brain in helping you to get thin.

CHAPTER 11

SLEEP YOUR WAY THIN

Principle: Sleep is necessary for your brain to be able to grow and function at optimal levels.

It's amazing what the right amount of sleep can do for you. You may have all the pieces in place to help you shed those pounds—you play and you exercise regularly—but without the right amount of sleep, there's a good chance that you won't be able to get to your desired weight. This is because sleep works to both rejuvenate your brain and help it to generate new and stronger connections. Achieving the loss of those unwanted pounds could be boosted by catching some ZZZs.

ONE SHEEP, TWO SHEEP

Knowing where you are when it comes to sleep will help you shape better habits to help you lose the weight, be healthy, and feel really good about yourself, so let's start off by taking a look at the quality and quantity of the rest you get every night.

The *How Rested Am I?* Quiz

1. The average amount of sleep I get each night is:

A. at least seven and a half hours.
B. between six and seven hours.
C. between four to six hours.
D. I'm supposed to sleep each night?

2. **When going to sleep each night, I:**

A. get right into bed, pull up the covers, and fall fast asleep.

B. read for a little bit in bed until I can fall asleep, which is usually within the hour.

C. fall asleep on the couch while watching the television.

D. lie in bed awake for hours, trying but unable to fall asleep.

3. **I nap for thirty minutes:**

A. nearly every day.

B. three to four days each week.

C. on weekend afternoons.

D. Naps? Why would I nap?

4. **I'm usually sleeping by:**

A. 9:30 P.M.

B. nearly midnight.

C. 2 A.M.

D. just as my alarm is about to go off.

5. **To me, a good night's sleep is:**

A. essential to my health.

B. something I know is good for me, but don't get as often as I should.

C. a necessary evil.

D. next to impossible.

6. **When I wake after dreaming, I:**

A. write everything down as soon as I wake up.

B. almost always forget what I was dreaming about, unfortunately, even if it was really neat.

C. find that I am screaming or shaking because it was a nightmare.

D. I can't even remember the last time I had a dream.

7. **When it comes to my bed:**

A. I have a comfortable, supportive mattress and comfortable pillows and I change my bedding regularly.

B. I have a comfortable mattress but I think I need new pillows and/or sheets.

C. I have a slight sagging area in my mattress and my pillows just aren't that comfortable anymore.

D. I sleep wherever I can find a cushion, and sometimes use a pillow and blanket.

8. **At the sound of the alarm going off in the morning, I:**

A. turn it off right away and am ready to go for the day.

B. turn it off, but lie there a few minutes until I feel a little more alert.

C. press the snooze button and doze back off . . . multiple times.

D. ignore it because I didn't get enough sleep the night before.

Answer Key

If you checked mostly As, you have a good understanding of just how important sleep is, which is why you work to get the right amount each night. Of course there is always room for improvement, and you can still work to better utilize the power of sleep.

If you checked mostly Bs, you are right at the border, getting almost the right amount of sleep to function at top notch, but you just aren't getting enough. A review of your sleeping habits will help you maximize your sleep patterns to give your brain the right amount of down time it needs to help you function optimally during the day.

If you checked mostly Cs, let's face it—you, along with 40 percent of Americans, just aren't getting enough sleep. Missing out on the right amount of sleep can have serious repercussions on your health, and it may be preventing you from maintaining a healthy weight without you even realizing it.

If you checked mostly Ds, it's no wonder you have a hard time with your weight—you're simply not getting enough sleep and the effects are controlling other aspects of your life. In fact, you may be among the roughly 70 million Americans that suffer from sleep disorders.

THE THREE RS OF SLEEP

From top to bottom, sleep allows your body to restore, renew, and reorganize itself. During the course of a good night's sleep, your cells will be able to repair themselves, your energy levels reload, and your mood stabilizes. Overall, sleep allows your body to recharge, which is good for your health. To really achieve the biggest benefit from sleep, you need anywhere from seven and a half to nine hours nightly; this is adequate time to recharge your body and allow it to lessen the damage placed on it by things like stress and harmful environmental exposures that you may come in contact with every day. Not to mention that getting enough sleep allows your body systems to regroup, getting you ready for the next day and boosting your energy level so that you wake up feeling energized and stay that way throughout the day. Why do we need this much sleep? It's because that is the time it takes for your body to head off into dreamland, which is where your brain kicks in and gets the chance to recharge.

Not getting enough sleep takes these benefits away from the body, leaving you feeling tired and groggy and focusing less on your health. Even worse, a lack of sleep really does negatively impact your health, which when coupled with excess weight, can greatly increase your risks of the following:

1. High blood pressure and cholesterol.
2. Putting your body on high alert, sending your blood pressure and your stress hormones way up. Chronic insomnia can result in a sustained hyperarousal state of your body's response system for stress, and this can add to problems controlling your weight.

3. Increasing stress hormones and inflammation in your body, both of which have negative health implications, like increasing your risk for certain chronic diseases (heart disease, cancer, diabetes).
4. Carrying around excess body fat, classifying you as overweight or obese. This is because two of the hormones involved in regulating hunger, ghrelin and leptin, are interrupted and unable to do their job properly when you don't get enough sleep.

Resting on a Healthy Weight

Studies consistently show that sleep is a vital component to managing your weight. One recent study conducted by Kaiser Permanente researchers showed that sleep is linked to obesity and weight problems. While the findings do not imply that poor sleep habits cause obesity or that good sleep habits result in weight loss, the underlying issue was that poor sleep can impact stress levels and this can influence your ability to eat right and exercise . . . even if you're making healthy choices throughout the day. Subjects in the study were given guidance on changing habits to be healthier, including a reduction in calorie intake coupled with a moderately intensive exercise plan. After six months, those participants getting between six and eight hours of sleep nightly had better success when it came to losing weight.

See, getting enough quality sleep really does have an impact on your health, and not just with your weight. One good way to maintain your weight and reduce your risk of developing chronic diseases is to get the right amount of sleep each night. Try it . . . your body will thank you!

LOSE SLEEP, KEEP THE WEIGHT

When you aren't getting enough sleep each night, you are setting yourself up for failure when it comes to losing the weight because it promotes:

- Lethargy, and general lack of motivation
- Irritability and mood swings
- A decrease in problem-solving skills
- Inability to deal well with stressful situations
- Indecisiveness

All in all, not getting enough sleep stops you from being in a positive mood, remaining stress free, and feeling confident in your decision-making skills—all of which are needed to help you live a healthy lifestyle. On the other hand, when you are well rested you have a better sense of what is going on, feel better about yourself and your decision-making skills, and can confidently make choices that are good for your health, and good for your waistline.

SEND YOUR BRAIN TOWARD SLEEP

Both your body and your brain need enough restful sleep each night, but not getting enough can wreak havoc on your brain. So, what exactly constitutes severe sleep deprivation? Severe sleep deprivation is not sleeping for three or four days, or having very erratic sleeping habits for a prolonged period of time. But even moderate sleep deprivation can be enough to slow down your brain. When your brain doesn't get the rest it needs, it is preventing neurons from being able to fire properly, derailing important circadian rhythms and even impairing neurogenesis. Sleep deprivation affects the ability to create new synapses and can limit the plasticity of your brain.

And it's not just your actual body that needs to get rest each night. Your brain also needs to get sleep. In fact, sleep is considered essential to a healthy brain; it allows it to function at its greatest potential and assists in myelin formation. Myelin is the layer surrounding nerves and insulating them, acting as a form of protection and also functional as well. Neurons need myelin to carry messages long distances in a short time. Getting enough sleep will also improve the ability of your brain to focus and help you retain important information.

YOUR GUIDE TO SLEEP

Once asleep, there are five stages you will cycle through every 90 to 110 minutes, including the deep restorative sleep and REM sleep stages, which are critical. Here are the stages:

Stage 1: **Transition to sleep.** This only lasts for about five minutes. Here we find that eye movements will slow, as will muscle activity. In addition, very slow theta waves are produced by the brain.

Stage 2: **Light sleep.** This stage lasts for ten to twenty-five minutes. Here we have slower brain waves interspersed with infrequent surges of accelerated brain waves called sleep spindles.

Stage 3: **Deep, restorative (slow-wave) sleep.** This stage is a transitional period between light sleep and deep sleep. Delta waves begin to appear.

Stage 4: **Delta sleep.** This a deep sleep that last for about 30 minutes and produces slow delta waves in the brain. This stage will shorten as the night goes on. It is in this phase that blood flow moves away from the brain and flows to the muscles.

Stage 5: **REM sleep.** We first see this occur at about seventy to ninety minutes after first falling asleep. This is the rapid eye movement (REM) phase where we see dreaming occur. The focus here is specifically on restoring the brain. The eye movements will become rapid, breathing becomes shallow, the limbs become temporarily paralyzed, and heart rate and blood pressure will increase. At this time, there will also be an increase in protein production. As the night goes on, the amount of time spent in REM sleep will increase.

As the night starts out, you spend a greater amount of time in Stages 3 and 4 of sleep, and less time in REM sleep. Then, as the night progresses, you shift away from the deep restorative sleep and start having more of the REM sleep. In the few hours just before waking, you will spend most of your time in stages 1, 2, and REM sleep, only briefly passing through the deep-sleep stages.

These stages of sleep play a role in how your brain and body recharge after your day. Without getting the right sleep in each stage you don't get those benefits of recharging and both your brain and body can suffer.

Sleep for Energy

Most research on sleep has been focused on the deep-sleep stages and how this benefits the body. Only recently has more focus moved to those earlier stages. It turns out that these stages really do deserve to be studied because they play an important role. In a Harvard Medical Research study that looked at rats during those early stages of sleep, results showed that the levels of adenosine triphosphate (ATP), which is the energy currency of cells in body, increase dramatically within four key brain regions; areas that are normally active during the awake state, particularly within the frontal cortex. This suggests that a rush of energy happens during the early sleep stages, which may be integral in replenishing brain functions that are essential to normal function in the awake state. If that is the case, then when your brain isn't passing through those early stages of sleep, it has to spend time the next day struggling to find energy. So make sure to get the sleep you need so you are rested and energetic come the next day.

Recharge Your Body

In the slow-wave or deep, restorative phase, the emphasis is on recharging your body, which is necessary to allow it to be restored and ready for the next day. This slow-wave sleep is also what sets the stage for REM sleep, which is needed to recharge your brain.

Recharge Your Brain

Once you enter into the REM phase, the focus moves from your body onto your brain. Your breathing becomes shallow, muscle activity slows down, and your heart and blood pressure will increase, all in an effort to allow your brain to be front and center and have a chance to recharge. It is important to have REM sleep because this is essential to learning and memory, both of which can help you in changing your habits to healthier ones. Rockefeller University researchers found that in rats those brain cells activated during awake times and also seem to reactivate during REM sleep, and this can help us better remember what we learned earlier that day.

Your brain does the following during REM sleep:

1. Consolidates and processes the information from everything you've learned throughout the day.
2. Forms neuronal connections that will strengthen and firm your newly made memories.
3. Replenishes neurotransmitters, including serotonin and dopamine, which are integral to helping all parts of the brain work at its maximum potential.

Moreover, sleep is also known to increase brain plasticity, which is important for helping you continue on learning as you get older.

Sleep to Remember!

Declarative memory is the memory of facts—what you ate for lunch, where you left your cell phone, and what you heard on the radio on the way to work. Harvard Medical School Division of Sleep Medicine professor Dr. Robert Stickgold completed a study on the effects of sleep on declarative memory. First, he taught two groups of people word pairs (two words to be remembered together, as a pair), and then sent one group to take a nap, while having the other group remain awake. After the napping group awoke, all participants were taught another set of word pairs, known as "interference" word pairs, with the purpose of confusing their memory of the original word pairings. Immediately following this, all participants were quizzed on their ability to recall the initial word pairs they were given. Those who were in the group that took a nap were better able to remember those initial word pairs. Approximately 76 percent were able to remember those words, while only 32 percent from the group that remained awake could remember those initial word pairs.

DREAM YOURSELF THIN

You may not realize it, but you typically spend greater than two hours of your sleep time dreaming each night. During the REM phase, a part of your brain known as the pons, which is located at the base of your brain, sends signals out to the thalamus. From there the messages are sent to the cortex, which is the outer layer of the brain that is involved with learning and organizing information. Scientists believe that the cortex works to interpret random signals that it receives from both the pons and the thalamus, and then pieces that information together to form a complete story.

Reaching a state of deep sleep promotes dreaming, and it is those dreams that aid the brain in processing the events that took place during the day. It is those dreams that allow your brain to form connections among sensory input, emotions, and memories.

GET THE SLEEP YOU NEED TO GET THIN

It is important to nurture deep restoration (slow-wave) sleep and REM (dreaming) sleep because both play a critical role in allowing your brain to properly process, retain, and integrate what happens when you are in the awake state. Allowing yourself to get the right amount of sleep will benefit your brain tremendously, allowing you to keep your brain pliable and functioning at its highest potential. In order to really get the sleep that you need to benefit your brain (and your body), you will need to stay away from things that interfere with your ability to fall asleep and stay that way. Here is what you should be doing and what you should avoid in order to improve your overall quality of sleep.

Unwind

Relaxation is critical to helping you get a good night's sleep. Exercise generally stimulates cortical alertness, which is not what you want when you are trying to get a restful night's sleep. Exercise does work to decrease stress, but intense aerobic exercise places your nervous system into a state of moderate arousal, which is not ideal when it comes time to go to sleep. Avoid exercising within two hours of heading to bed. If this is the only time you have for intense exercise, consider having a light snack after your workout to help maintain blood sugars and prevent you from having trouble sleeping due to hunger.

Abstain

Alcohol has many effects on the body, and one of these is the reduction of time spent in REM sleep. There is a cumulative effect here, so the more you consume, the less time you will spend in REM sleep, and this translates to feeling less rested when you wake up. If you do decide to drink alcohol before bed, make sure to leave at least one hour for the body to process the alcohol before heading off to sleep. Also, don't forget to drink some water since alcohol dehydrates the body.

Eat Lightly

For the most part, you need to be energized in the morning and afternoon hours, not at night, so larger meals should come earlier in the day. Eating a big meal during the evening hours means that your digestive system is put to work, which can interfere with sleep—particularly the deeper phases. While there is no science behind the tales of not eating after 7 or 8 P.M. to lose weight, you will probably find it easier to sleep if you avoid heavy meals within two hours of sleeping. You will also want to avoid fatty and spicy foods before bed since both can interfere with a good night's sleep.

Bedtime Snack?

When it comes to weight loss, eating smaller, more frequent meals is best; this means it may be helpful to have a bedtime snack. Everyone will have different times that they go to sleep, so there is no magic number for what time to have this snack, but when it comes to comfort and quality of sleep, aim for one to two hours before bed. When selecting a bedtime snack, go with something low fat, containing some carbohydrates (aim for whole grains), and also some protein. Foods with the amino acid tryptophan—such as poultry, spinach, eggs, and dairy products—can also be beneficial for getting you off to dreamland.

Stick to a Schedule

Getting on a sleep schedule is important, but don't forget that this also applies to weekends, not just weekdays. This shows your brain and your body that there are certain times designated to sleep and other times meant for being awake. On the other hand, if you find that you are chronically not getting enough sleep, it may actually be a good idea to use the weekends to catch up on sleep. Dr. David Dinges, chief of the Division of Sleep and Chronobiology at the University of Pennsylvania, conducted a study that demonstrated the benefits of one long night of sleep (ten hours) in otherwise healthy adult subjects. The results even showed that this extended sleep for one night was enough to boost performance to roughly the same level of people who were getting ten hours of sleep every night during the week. Of course this can be beneficial to help you catch up on some much-needed sleep, but remember that when it comes to losing weight, you may want to swap out those lazy Sundays in bed for something that burns more energy.

Create a Welcoming Sleep Environment

Your sleep environment really makes a difference in your ability to fall asleep and stay that way. Aim for a temperature somewhere between 68°F and 72°F and be sure to close your curtains or blinds to keep out the light. Lastly, make sure to cut out any noise or other distractions, like the television.

Bring It Down a Notch

Create a sense of relaxation before bed by participating in stress-reducing activities that promote relaxation, such as meditation or slow stretching with deep breathing. Avoid things like starting to work on a complicated project, reading intense books, or watching violent movies or television shows. Instead, pick activities that are restful and help you bring down your stress levels before bed.

Make a Bedtime Routine

Just like telling a child a story every night to help put him or her to sleep, you can benefit from a nightly, bedtime routine. Curling up in bed with a lighthearted book may be just what you need. Or maybe writing about your day in a journal will help you release any last bits of stress from the day. Whatever routine you pick, make sure it is something that will relax you, and then do this for ten minutes every night before drifting off to sleep.

Avoid Caffeine

Coffee, sodas, energy drinks, and any other food or drink that contains caffeine can prevent you from getting the sleep you need. Not to mention the fact that some of those may also contain calories that will sabotage your plans to lose weight. There are some hidden sources of caffeine out there, too (like chocolate, some noncola sodas, and some pain relievers), so make sure to check what you're eating and drinking before bed—including your medicines.

Try Warm Milk

Adding extra calories in is not always the best idea when trying to lose weight, but there are some benefits to drinking milk if you are having trouble sleeping. Milk contains L-tryptophan, an amino acid and precursor of melatonin and serotonin, both of which promote sleep. Aim for 4 ounces of fat-free or 1 percent milk if you find that milk does the trick and lulls you off to sleep.

Reduce Stress

The trick to getting a good night's sleep may be as simple as reducing stress. Take some time before bed to chill out. The 2007 Stress and Anxiety Disorders survey conducted by the Anxiety Disorders Association of America found that, of those adults who suffer from stress-induced sleep difficulties, three fourths report that this lack of sleep increased their stress levels during the day. This means there may be more stress later on, which won't help you to break the cycle and get the sleep that you need. In addition, stress makes it hard to make healthy decisions during the day and can increase hormones that make it hard to lose the weight. Cutting back on stress will help you sleep better and allow you to wake up refreshed and ready to face the day with a positive attitude and a readiness to make the right choices to lose the weight and keep you healthy.

Meditation Can Improve Well-Being and Promote Weight Loss Success

A 2011 study published in the *International Journal of Obesity* looked at weight loss and the links between obesity and hours of sleep and stress levels. Those participants who had the least amount of stress and slept from six to eight hours nightly were more likely to lose weight than the others. Getting the right amount of sleep and reducing your stress may be key elements in managing your weight, not to mention they can help you stay alert and focused during the day, allowing you to make wiser decisions. Moreover, the researchers indicated that if you have trouble sleeping or find yourself stressed out often, meditation may be just the technique you need to help you out.

GOOD DREAMS, GOOD FIGURE

Remember, sleep is just as good for your figure as it is for your brain because it:

- Promotes your health and well-being.
- Allows you to have the time needed for your body and brain to restore, repair, and regenerate.
- Boosts your mood, creates a positive outlook, and increases your energy level.
- Helps you to better handle the normal stress that comes up in everyday life.
- Helps your brain to expand and master new skills.

Train your brain to get the rest it needs and you'll be operating at peak levels to achieve your goals and lose the pounds. So grab your pillow, release the day's stress, and sweet dreams to you!

CHAPTER 12

EAT YOUR WAY THIN

Principle: Your brain depends upon your ability to fuel it with the nutrients it needs to optimally function.

You probably already know that what you eat is essential for your health, your energy level, and how much you weigh, but the importance of nutrition goes beyond just powering your body. Good nutrition is essential to having a brain that works for you—not against you—when it comes to getting to the healthy weight you desire and it is important that you nourish that brain well. Although your brain comprises around 2 percent of your total body weight, it uses up a disproportionate amount of your resources: 20 percent of your body's blood supply, 20 percent of its oxygen supply, and 65 percent of its glucose supply. This means that, overall, a lot of your daily nutrition is put toward supporting a healthy brain. In this chapter you will learn about the important changes that you need to make to your diet and foods and info on what you should be eating regularly to provide good nutrition, both for your brain and your body.

NOURISH YOUR BRAIN

While you may often hear the word *diet* used in a negative way, or a way that makes you cringe, the real, deep-down meaning of the word (and a much more positive one) is anything that you eat or drink for nourishment. Eating the right diet to provide your brain with the nutrients it needs also ensures that you are eating the right diet to manage your weight . . . assuming you are staying within your caloric needs. Before we discuss specific nutrient needs, let's take a quick inventory of your current eating habits and see if you are feeding your brain well.

The *Feed Your Brain* Quiz

1. You apply the USDA's meal planning guidelines, MyPlate, at:

A. every meal you eat.

B. most of the meals you eat.

C. when the foods you want fit those guidelines.

D. Whose plate?

2. For breakfast, you eat:

A. whole grain cereal, low-fat milk, and a piece of fruit.

B. bacon and eggs.

C. doughnuts or a pastry.

D. I'm not a breakfast person.

3. You eat from fast-food establishments:

A. No way! I never eat fast food.

B. for a special treat.

C. a few times each week.

D. at least one meal every day.

4. When it comes to dietary fats, you:

A. eat heart healthy unsaturated fats, including omega-3 fatty acids.

B. stick with "good" fats.

C. avoid eating trans fats.

D. don't really care about the kind of fat, just as long as the food tastes good.

5. **Your protein comes primarily from:**
   A. low-fat dairy, fish, and legumes (beans).
   B. fish and white-meat chicken.
   C. meat.
   D. sausage, bacon, or hot dogs.

6. **The vegetable you eat most often is:**
   A. anything dark green.
   B. whatever is on sale or fits in my budget.
   C. tomatoes on my sandwich.
   D. french fries.

Answer Key

If you checked mostly As, you have a good understanding that you have to do more than just feed your body. You also need to feed your brain as well for it to perform optimally. Good nutrition and eating right is tough, so there is always room to improve your diet to maximize your brainpower while shedding those pounds.

If you checked mostly Bs, you know that some foods are better choices than others but you still need to focus on what will not only help maintain your weight, but also best fuel your brain. Improving your nutrition intake will allow your brain to work better, helping you stay focused on making better choices and leading a healthy life.

If you checked mostly Cs, your uncertainty toward nutrition is not only impacting your weight, but also impacting the function of your brain. Knowing what you should eat for brain health will translate to knowing what—and how much—to eat to get you to a healthy weight.

If you checked mostly Ds, your lack of education about proper eating is keeping your weight steady or climbing, and your brain is suffering the consequences, making it harder than ever for you to change your lifestyle habits and shed those pounds. Adjusting your eating habits will not only impact your weight right off the bat, but the improvement to your brain function will also help you maintain the healthy weight you desire.

Eating the right foods to fuel your brain also provides your body overall with the nutrition it needs; so as long as you are eating the right amount of calories, you will be able to lose the weight and keep it off. The foods that provide your brain with the essential vitamins and minerals it needs will also provide those same nutrients to your body. This will help keep your nutrition up, while preventing you from eating the foods that will slow your body down and pack on the pounds.

Early Signs from Your Brain

When you aren't eating well and getting the right nutrients, signs of malnutrition may be the first warning signs that something isn't right. A change in mental status could be an indicator that you are deficient in a nutrient or that your diet isn't well balanced. Actually, this early warning sign comes from your brain because the frontal lobes are sensitive to dropping glucose levels. Glucose is the primary source of energy that fuels the brain, so when you don't get enough, your brain signals emergency mode. Symptoms of low glucose levels include mood swings, irritability, and generally just being in a bad mood. Other brain areas affected are those that regulate vital functions like breathing and heart rhythm. It is not uncommon for people trying to lose weight to cut back on eating and go too long between meals—maybe even cutting carbohydrate intake dangerously low—so if someone mentions your mood and personality seem a little off, maybe a little grumpy, consider having a small snack with healthy whole grains to raise your glucose levels.

THE BASICS OF HEALTHY EATING

The more you know about nutrition, the better—but you don't need to be a trained expert to understand the basic principles and know enough to keep you lean and healthy. Some foods are better than others, and this depends on the amount of desirable nutrients they provide per serving. Some foods that provide a lot of good nutrients for a small amount of calories include:

- Fruits and vegetables in a variety of colors, which are packed with antioxidants and fiber.
- Whole-grain, fiber-filled foods like brown rice, whole-wheat bread, whole-wheat pasta, oats, barley, and quinoa (there are many others).
- Lean proteins, like fish, white-meat poultry, lean cuts of meat, legumes, eggs, low-fat dairy, and soy.
- Omega-3 fatty acids, found in fish, flaxseed oil, canola oil, soybeans, pumpkin seeds, and walnuts.
- Nutrient-rich foods, which are those foods packed with many vitamins and minerals in each serving.

Other foods (those you should eat less often) provide very few of the nutrients you need and contain a larger number of calories. Foods to avoid include:

- Saturated fats, found in fatty cuts of red meat, cheese, full-fat dairy products, and fried food.
- Trans fats, which are formed when oils are altered to be solid and can be found in margarines, many baked goods (especially if they are not homemade), and fast food.
- Refined grains like white rice, white bread, and "wheat" bread that is not 100 percent whole grain.

- Nutrient-poor foods, which are those that are high in calories per serving but don't provide many desirable nutrients and often contain added saturated fats and sugars.
- Overly processed, prepackaged foods containing added saturated fats and sugars.
- High-sodium foods.
- Beverages with added sugars—particularly sodas and some juices—as these pack in the calories but not the vitamins and minerals (and you won't get the benefit of fiber when drinking juice).

And, while everyone needs a different amount of calories each day, the basic nutrition guidelines *guide* you toward making the best choices within your own caloric needs.

According to the data compiled by the United States Department of Agriculture (USDA), Americans overdo it when it comes to saturated fats and added sugars, consuming—on average—35 percent of their total calories from those sources. The recommendation is to keep the intake of saturated fats and added sugars to only 5 to 15 percent of total calories for most people each day.

WHAT TO PUT ON YOUR PLATE

Do you remember the pyramid figure used to represent the food groups and healthy eating patterns? Well, in 2011 that classic pyramid was replaced with the MyPlate. This is a visual representation of the USDA guidelines for general nutrition that serves as a guidance tool to help Americans make their food choices, pointing them in the direction of healthy foods. Key components of MyPlate—and any healthy diet—include variety, balance, and moderation. The amount of food you need daily from each of the food groups really depends on individual characteristics like age, gender, and activity level. Below we've provided you with the general guidelines for adults. For more detailed information visit the website at *www.MyPlate.gov*.

While the presentation of a healthy diet has changed from a pyramid to a plate, the food groups themselves remain the same and include the following:

- **Grains:** Select whole grains and products made from whole grains. Aim to fill roughly 25 to 30 percent of your plate with grains, which for adults is about 6 to 8 ounces of grains per day. Look for whole grains and make half your daily intake of grains from whole grains. Aim for whole grains! Look for the words "whole grain" or "100 percent whole grain" on the label, and you can also use the Whole Grains Stamp for help determining if you have selected a whole-grain product. A bonus to eating whole grains is that they are packed with fiber, which helps to keep you feeling fuller between meals.
- **Vegetables:** Aim to fill around 30 percent of your plate with vegetables. Make sure to get a variety of vegetables, including those that are green and those that are red- and orange-colored. Don't forget that frozen vegetables will provide you with good nutrients, just like fresh.
- **Fresh fruits:** Aim to fill around 20 percent of your plate with fruits, and in general always aim to make half your plate filled with fruits and vegetables. To help manage your weight, stick with whole fruits and avoid juices, especially those with added sugar.
- **Dairy:** It's not located on the plate, but that doesn't mean it isn't part of a healthy diet. You can find the milk pictured as a glass next to your plate. You want to aim for low-fat dairy products. Whole milk is not recommended over age two due to the fat content, which also impacts the calorie content. The goal is to aim for three cups of milk per day, but this can come from yogurt and other low-fat dairy products as well. The focus with the dairy group is the calcium. But don't worry if you can't tolerate milk due to lactose intolerance or a milk protein allergy,

or if you choose to not drink it because you are a vegetarian; there are other nondairy ways to get your calcium in each day.

- **Protein-Filled Foods:** This includes meat, poultry, fish, dry beans, eggs, nuts, and meat substitutes. Aim to fill around 20 percent of your plate with protein-filled foods, focusing on those that are lean and low in fat. Avoid processed meats that have added sodium. Most adults need between 5 and 6 ounces of lean protein each day, but that can vary from person to person. The Recommended Dietary Allowance (RDA) for protein is 0.8 grams per kilogram of body weight. The total needs for the day will include protein grams coming from these protein-filled foods and the protein coming from the other food groups, like dairy and vegetables.

Sweets and fats are not a focus on MyPlate, and these are the foods to limit each day. One thing to remember is that there are heart-healthy fats, like those in olive oil, avocado, and nuts, and these are a healthy addition to the diet. Just watch your portions because the calories in fats add up fast—so you don't want to eat too many servings. The fats to cut back on are those in cakes, candies, cookies, and other "sweets," and those in fried and fast foods.

What's a Serving?

This is an area of confusion among many people. It is not uncommon to overestimate your portions when trying to match these up with what really equals one serving. With the increase in portions from restaurants, it is getting harder and harder to tell how much we should be eating at one time. Let's take a look at some basic serving sizes for foods in each of the food groups.

- One serving of grains: 1 slice of bread; 1 ounce of ready-to-eat cereal; ½ cup of cooked whole-grain cereal, rice, or pasta
- One serving of vegetables: 1 cup of raw leafy vegetables; ½ cup of other vegetables, cooked or chopped raw; ¾ cup of vegetable juice

- One serving of fruit: 1 medium piece of fruit (for example: apple, banana, or orange); ½ cup of chopped, cooked, or canned fruit (look for those canned in water or their own juices); ¾ cup fruit juice
- One serving of dairy (1 cup equivalent): 1 cup of milk or yogurt; 1½ ounces of hard cheese; 2 ounces of processed cheese (American); ⅓ cup of shredded cheese; ½ cup ricotta cheese
- One serving of a protein food (1 ounce equivalent): 1 ounce of cooked lean meat, poultry, or fish; ½ cup of cooked beans; 1 tablespoons of peanut- or other nut butter; 1 ounce of nuts; 2 ounces of tofu; 1 egg

It's a good idea to keep these serving sizes in mind because what you may find on the food label of a product as the serving is just what the food company calls a serving. This may turn out to be more than what is truly considered one serving from the food group, and can result in overeating.

What about Calories?

While it's important to get the right kind of calories to give your brain what it needs, it is just as important when managing your weight to make sure that those calories are not exceeding what your body needs each day. A calorie is a unit of measurement that relates to the amount of heat released from foods. Everyone has different needs for calories daily, and these can change depending on activity levels.

These are the general guidelines from the USDA, which are really just a guide or place for you to start before making the adjustments you need to manage your weight, and are determined based on someone who is not physically active: the recommendation for females nineteen to thirty years of age is 2,000 calories; for males nineteen to thirty years of age, 2,400 calories; for females thirty-one to fifty years of age, 1,800 calories; for males thirty-one to fifty years of age, 2,200 calories.

Again, each person's caloric needs will depend on things like height, weight, age, and activity level. Since the goal is to train your brain to get thin, it's important to remember that your brain can't do *all* the work, and calories do matter when it comes to managing your weight. You should have an idea of the range to aim for each day, and allow your brain to help you make the right choices to fill those calories each day. One of the common equations used, which accounts for obesity, is the Mifflin-St. Jeor equation. To calculate your own needs, you will need to find your height in centimeters and your weight in kilograms:

Male: BMR = (10 × weight) + (6.25 × height) – (5 × age) + 5

Female: BMR = (10 × weight) + (6.25 × height) – (5 × age) – 161

Once you have the BMR, which stands for Basal Metabolic Rate, you will want to multiple by an activity factor:

1.200 = sedentary (little or no exercise)

1.375 = lightly active (light exercise/sports one to three days per week)

1.550 = moderately active (moderate exercise/sports three to five days per week)

1.725 = very active (hard exercise/sports six to seven days per week)

1.900 = extra active (very hard exercise/sports and physical job)

Once you have multiplied the BMR by one of these factors you have a number that represents the predicted amount of calories you need each day. Of course this is only an estimate, but this is the best place to start. Also, keep in mind this is just a single number, so you may find that some days you are just above this number and other days you are a little below this number. That's to be expected. Remember that your body has the ultimate say as to whether you are eating the right amount of calories. If you notice that you are gaining weight, then your estimated calorie number is too high and you should decrease this because you are really working to lose weight. If you notice that with that number you are maintaining your weight, you will also want to decrease your calorie goals because your plan is to lose weight. It is a little more complex to determine how much to decrease this number by each day, but on average, 500 calories will result in around a pound of weight loss per week, so with no changes in your exercise plans, this may be the best number with which to start.

SUGAR WARS

You know sugar isn't good for your health, but did you know that it's not good for your brain either? At the Salk Institute in California, researchers noted that sugar damaged cells all over the body, particularly in the brain. Also, University of Wisconsin researchers found that the brain may have a similar reaction to too many refined added sugars, just as it would if it were a virus or bacteria, resulting in an immune response, which can then lead to cognitive deficits, similar to those seen in people with Alzheimer's disease. In addition, excessive consumption of refined added sugars can:

- Block cellular membranes, resulting in slower neural communication.
- Increase inflammation in your brain.
- Increase levels of stress hormone cortisol, leading to memory impairment.
- Impair synaptic communication.
- Cause neurons to misfire and send inaccurate messages, wasting the time and energy of your brain trying to make sense of them.
- Increase delta, alpha, and theta brain waves, which are all the slower brain waves. This can make it harder to clearly process information coming in to your brain.

Over time, doing all of these things can damage your neurons.

Give Up the Soda

It's no surprise that soda is bad for your health. The empty calories add up quickly and it doesn't do much to curb your appetite. But besides the general weight-related reason to pass on the soda, there are also the brain-related reasons. Glucose, the version of sugar that your body uses for energy, is the main supply of energy utilized by your brain. However, having too much or too little glucose can negatively impact your brain function. Just one soda can provide you with the same amount of glucose as 10 teaspoons of table sugar. That's a lot of sugar coming into your bloodstream at one time considering the normal amount in your blood stream is around the amount found in 4 teaspoons of sugar. To compensate for the sudden rush of sugar, your pancreas releases a lot of insulin, all in an effort to bring your blood sugar back into the normal range. Some sugar makes it into your cells, including brain cells, and then the rest will be stored for energy use later (including stored as fat). About an hour later, your blood sugar, still feeling the effects of all that insulin released, may drop and result in a low blood sugar. The constant ups and downs are not only harmful to your health, but can also result in impaired memory and foggy thought patterns.

HOLD THE SALT

There is some evidence that having too much sodium can cause a stroke, but there are certainly more factors that play into increasing your risk including other modifiable factors like obesity and physical activity level. Since high blood pressure is a risk factor for stroke, watching your sodium intake will not only benefit your health in general, but can also lower your risk for stroke—ultimately benefiting your brain.

The previous Dietary Guidelines for Americans called for a daily sodium intake of 2,400 mg. Recently this was lowered to 1,500 mg for a few groups of people, including people who are over fifty-one years of age, African Americans (who have an increased risk for high blood pressure), and those who already have high blood pressure, renal failure (chronic), or diabetes. Of course, cutting back on sodium can be beneficial to everyone, especially if you are looking to lose weight, because sodium plays a role in fluid balance in the body. Too much sodium can lead to the body retaining fluid, which in turns leads to a bloated feeling and excess weight to carry around. In order to get rid of some of the excess sodium in your diet, avoid frequent consumption of prepackaged/prepared meals, cured meats, cheeses, many canned goods, pickles, most soups, soy sauce, and mustard. There are other foods like these, so always make sure to check the nutrition label on your foods to see how much sodium a food contains per serving. To cut back on sodium but still enjoy soups and canned vegetables, look for products listed as low sodium or no added salt. You will still want to check the label for the sodium content, but there is a good chance it will be lower than the "regular" product. You can also cut down your sodium intake by not adding salt to your food at the table and using herbs and spices to flavor foods when cooking at home.

Why Getting a B Is a Good Thing

The B might as well stand for "Brain." The B vitamins (1, 2, 3, 6, and 12) are a set of compounds that you need to get from your diet, and all play a role in brain health. It's very important to make sure that you get all of the B vitamins, and not just focus on one over another. They all work together to help boost your brain function. As an added bonus, they also play a role in metabolizing carbohydrates, fats, and proteins, and help your body best use the energy you provide it with the foods you eat. This means you will be better able to metabolize the carbohydrates and provide your brain with the fuel it needs. In addition, B vitamins help improve mood and produce neurotransmitters. People who are deficient in B vitamins tend to have an increased risk for depression and anxiety, along with other brain-related conditions like memory loss and abnormal brain waves.

START YOUR DAY OFF RIGHT

There's a reason why people say breakfast is the most important meal of the day, and although all meals are important and contribute to good health, breakfast really does get you off to the right start. When you wake up in the morning, your body has been in a fasting state overnight and eating breakfast helps to boost your glucose stores, sending some much-needed fuel to your brain and setting you up for clear thinking during the day. Not only does this benefit your brain, but it also helps manage your weight since eating breakfast is linked with weight loss. Of the weight loss maintainers who provided their weight loss data to the National Weight Control Registry, 78 percent reported eating breakfast every day. This is one habit that will help you achieve your *thin* weight.

Need some breakfast ideas? Try these suggestions:

- Fortified breakfast cereals (not heavily sweetened) with sliced fruit and fat-free milk
- A whole-grain waffle topped with 1 tablespoon of nut butter and ½ banana
- Two tablespoons of peanut- or almond butter on a whole-wheat bagel
- Cottage cheese and pineapple
- Oatmeal with dried fruits and nuts
- A vegetable-filled egg-white omelet with one slice whole-grain bread, toasted
- A hard-boiled egg, a piece of fruit, and a slice of whole-grain bread
- Low-fat or nonfat Greek yogurt with fruit

No matter what healthy foods you choose for breakfast, you are taking a step in the right direction by adding this meal into your healthy lifestyle.

Catch the Bad Guys

Free radicals are unstable atoms with an electron missing, and can roam your body causing damage that has been linked to cancer development and heart disease. Fortunately, antioxidants are substances that stop free radicals from causing damage by stabilizing them. This means that antioxidants are a desirable part of your dietary intake because free radicals can build up in the brain faster than any other area of your body. In order to benefit from powerful antioxidants like vitamin C or lycopene, follow the MyPlate guidelines and fill half your plate with fruits and vegetables. Aim for dark greens and strive for fall colors (reds, yellows, and oranges). Even purple and blue produce packs an antioxidant punch.

FAT IS GOOD

Fats play a role in carrying, absorbing, and storing the fat-soluble vitamins (A, D, E, and K). Around 60 percent of your brain is composed of fats, and they are part of *all* cell membranes. However, not all fats are created equal—and the type you eat really makes a difference. A diet packed with saturated fats (the bad fats) will not only promote the development of heart disease, but your brain will only be able to make low-quality cell membranes, impacting the ability of neurons to function properly. On the other hand, a diet containing unsaturated fats (the good fats) will help keep your heart healthy and allow your brain cells to produce higher-quality cell membranes, ultimately helping your neurons function at optimal levels. Fat grams pack just over twice the amount of calories found in one gram of carbohydrate or protein, and these can add up fast. Unfortunately, it is possible to overdo it, even when you're eating something healthy, so watch how much fat you're eating, and make sure that only around 30 percent of your total daily calories are coming from fats. Good sources of fats include oils (like olive and canola), avocado, nuts, and fatty fish (like salmon and mackerel).

Give Flax a Chance

To boost your ability to focus, give flax a chance. Remember—when it comes to flax, oils or ground flaxseeds are the way to go (the whole seeds may not provide the same benefit). Try adding either to baked goods to increase your flax intake. Or add some to hot cereal or yogurt. Flax is an excellent source of alpha-linolenic acid (ALA), which is one of the omega-3 fatty acids. It helps improve the function of the cerebral cortex, which is the area of the brain involved in processing sensory information.

Omega-3s, Please

As we mentioned before, there are some fats that are good for you, and omega-3 fatty acids fall into this category. Just like other fats, they are calorie dense—but they provide benefits to your health, which means that eating foods with omega-3s in the right amounts will have positive results on your brain health. Currently, research is taking place to see if these essential fatty acids play a role in lowering the risk of dementia and Alzheimer's disease. These are some omega-3 fatty acid containing foods to include in your diet:

- Some fatty, coldwater fish (like salmon, herring, sardines, mackerel, rainbow trout, tuna, and whitefish)
- Canola oil
- Flaxseed oil
- Ground flaxseeds
- Walnuts

Omega-3 fatty acids are great for mental function, including clarity in thoughts, concentration, and the ability to focus, making these a good choice not only for adults but also for children. Unfortunately, the typical American child's diet contains few omega-3 fatty acids, so adding more to your diet may help increase omega 3 intake in your kids' lives too.

Mental Challenge Coming Up?

If you happen to have a mental challenge on the horizon, remember that B vitamins, such as folic acid, B_{12}, and B_6 play a role in helping messages to be carried back and forth between your brain and body. When you're eating meals and snacks with foods containing B vitamins, stick to foods over supplements if you can because you get a greater benefit (and possibly better absorption) when you get those nutrients from foods—particularly when those foods also contain other nutrients that will benefit you. Try out a small portion of seafood and leafy dark-green vegetables to help you stay focused. Or perhaps a bowl of whole-grain cereal, low-fat or fat-free milk, and a sliced egg is more up your alley to get your mental state in tip-top shape. Some other good brainpower boosters are bananas, nuts, and seeds.

Hold the Bad Fats

While good fats have positive effects on your brain and help keep you healthy, there is another group of fats that does just the opposite. Unfortunately, the typical American diet is higher in those bad, or unhealthy, fats than in those considered the good fats. These bad fats include saturated fats, which have been linked to heart disease, and are typically found in foods that pack a lot of calories with few vitamins and minerals. Unhealthy fats also include trans fats, which result from a process known as hydrogenation. This technique takes oils and makes them solid increasing their shelf-life, but in the process, the structure of these fats ends up promoting heart disease. You can find both of these kinds of unhealthy fats listed on the nutrition facts panel on packaged foods. These fats are solid—your healthy oils are liquid. Guidelines for saturated fats are to keep your consumption to less than 10 percent of your daily calorie intake. Saturated and trans fats can be found in:

- Many prepackaged, highly processed foods, including commercial baked goods, crackers, chips, and candy.
- Fast foods.
- Fatty cuts of red meat, dark meat chicken (and the skin).
- Full-fat dairy products including butter, whole milk, ice cream, and cheese (most margarines, as well, although those are dairy free).
- Some salad dressings.
- Coconut and palm oils.

Unlike healthy fats, trans fatty acids (you can spot them on the food label and listed on the ingredient list as "partially hydrogenated oils") become rigid as a result of the chemical structure, and can get in the way of proper synaptic or electrical nerve cell communication. Because these foods often contain lots of calories (not just from fat—they often have added sugar too) but very little nutritional benefit, trans fats can thwart your weight loss efforts. They can also:

- Modify the production of neurotransmitters, such as dopamine.
- Boost ldl (bad) cholesterol levels, while lowering hdl (good) cholesterol levels.
- Increase plaque build up in blood vessels, which increases the likelihood of blood clots forming, putting both your heart and brain at risk and leading to serious long-term health consequences.

- Interfere with energy production in the mitochondria (the energy factories) of brain cells.
- Raise triglyceride levels in your blood, which may slow down the amount of oxygen getting to your brain.

Keeping your diet free (or at least as low as possible) from trans fats benefits you in many ways. You will wind up eliminating many foods from your diet that provide little nutritional benefit and at the same time you'll keep yourself free from the negative effects that trans fats have on the brain and body.

CAFFEINE WAKE-UP CALL

It may seem like a good idea to get in oodles of caffeine daily, in order to help you stay awake and alert. In fact, you may have even heard that this can help you lose weight. In reality, there is no "miracle cure" here, and too much caffeine can damage your stomach, induce headaches, promote anxiety, and prevent you from getting a good night's sleep. We usually think of coffee right away when thinking about sources of caffeine, but it is important to mention that caffeine is also found in tea leaves and cocoa beans, and products made from these sources. Other hidden sources that you may not have realized include more than a thousand different over-the-counter and prescription drugs, and even decaffeinated coffee contains a very small amount. When it comes to your brain, caffeine may improve your level of alertness but research shows that it won't help if you need to use abstract thinking. And, as far as weight loss is concerned, caffeine may boost metabolism for a bit and shed some water weight, but there is not any strong scientific evidence to show that this is dramatic enough to make an impact on your weight long term, and it certainly does not outweigh the risks associated with excessive consumption of caffeine.

Caffeine Allowance

If your diet contains enough healthy beverages, such as water first and foremost, and perhaps some low-fat or fat-free milk, there is room for you to enjoy some coffee without feeling guilty. The pharmacological active dose for caffeine is listed at 200 milligrams, and the daily recommendation for intake suggests not exceeding the amount in one to three cups of coffee daily (139 to 417 milligrams). Not sure how much caffeine is found in some common caffeine-containing foods and beverages? Here is a list to help:

- 6 ounces of brewed coffee = 100 milligrams
- 6 ounces of tea brewed from whole leaves = 10–50 milligrams
- 12 ounces of cola = 50 milligrams
- 1 ounce of cocoa (like a milk chocolate bar) = 6 milligrams
- 1 cup of semisweet chocolate chips = 92 milligrams

See, just like with so many things in our lives, moderation plays a key role. Some caffeine can fit easily into a healthy life, and knowing how much is found in the foods and beverages you consume each day will help you make sure you aren't consuming too much.

Don't Send the Coffee Back Just Yet

A major protective feature of our brain is the "blood-brain barrier," which is a thin coating that keeps the brain separate from the rest of the body. This coating can become weakened and damaged from stress and disease. Recently researchers have found some evidence that caffeine, like that found in coffee products, could play a role in protecting the barrier and may repair the damage. So it looks like a cup of coffee may not be so bad after all—just don't take this to the extreme and use it as a free pass to have too much caffeine daily.

FOOD FOR LOSERS

It may not be the most scientific of terms, but there are some foods that really do deserve to be called *superfoods*, because they provide your body with a lot of the nutrients you need without giving you a lot of calories or things you don't need (like artery-clogging fats). In the end, all the foods you eat together impact your brain health and your weight, but a healthy diet full of a variety of superfoods will ensure that you are eating right to maintain your weight, prevent disease, and let your brain function optimally. Remember, having a healthy brain that lets you think clearly will pave the way for you to make healthy lifestyle choices.

It's Berry, Berry Good

Blueberries top the list when it comes to providing your brain with protection. Those pretty blue-colored berries are brimming with antioxidant and anti-inflammatory compounds, which have been found in some studies to have the potential to reverse short-term memory loss and slow down the aging process. Research on flavonoids, compounds that are found in blueberries, has been positive so far in showing benefits such as slowing mental decline, and the thought behind this is that flavonoids interact with the proteins found as part of the brain structure, positively impacting the function of the brain.

While many foods offer up antioxidants, blueberries have a leg up on some of the competition, providing 38 percent more antioxidants than red wine. These berries also come out on top when compared with other fruits and vegetables—plus they taste good, which alone should be enough to entice you to add some to your diet. Blueberries are in season (meaning they are generally cheaper at the grocery store) from around late May through the end of summer, but even when they aren't in season you can still enjoy them since they are sold frozen in most grocery stores. Try them in your oatmeal, on a salad, or tossed in Greek yogurt.

But not only blueberries contain flavonoids, so don't pass up other berries and fruits. Flavonoids are antioxidants, and are also found in foods like soy, green tea, and cherries. The foods that are most potent when it comes to flavonoids are those boasting red and purple hues. Some other berries not to be missed are goji berries, cranberries, blackberries, mulberries, cranberries, and boysenberries, all of which are filled with antioxidants and good for your brain. Variety is essential to enjoying your healthy diet, so don't forget to change up your berry lineup from time to time.

Nothing Fishy Going on Here

Fish is often touted as a superfood, and with good reason. Many fish are filled with omega-3 fatty acids. When coupled with nutrients like protein, vitamins, and minerals they put in overtime for your brain and your body. In the Hordaland Health Study in Norway, a sample of just over 2,000 elderly Norwegians, aged seventy to seventy-four, found that the subjects who ate any kind of fish were more likely to score better on cognitive tests than those who did not eat fish, and this was even after accounting for education level.

The American Heart Association recommends eating two three-and-a-half-ounce servings of fish weekly, particularly the fatty fish. Of course, there is some concern when it comes to fish and seafood—some are high in mercury, a toxin that can harm the brain. When it comes to eating fish, the best practice is to eat enough to have a benefit from the positive aspects of fish, but not so much as to have a problem with the many environmental toxins that can be found in fish. Watch your intake of species that are higher in mercury including shark, king mackerel, swordfish, and tilefish. The top performers when it comes to low mercury and high omega-3 content include Albacore tuna, sardines, salmon, mackerel, lake trout, and herring.

For your waistline, make sure you are keeping these healthy fish as a healthy part of your diet. The preparation of these foods will make a difference, so aim for grilling, broiling, poaching, or baking, rather than frying your fish. Look for low-sodium marinades, sauces, and seasonings. For a healthy meal, enjoy your fish with some vegetables and a whole grain.

Get Wild

There is no denying that salmon is a superior choice when it comes to your brain. However, not all salmon are raised equal. Your best bet, when it comes to getting those omega 3s without the possibility of antibiotics and with fewer environmental toxins, is wild salmon. Most of the time Atlantic salmon will be farmed, so look for Pacific kinds and check to see if it is wild salmon. Just remember that this can get pricey, so it doesn't need to be the only fish in your diet. Variety works too when it comes to fish and omega-3s. Looking to cut down on costs? Try canned varieties of wild salmon.

Queen Quinoa

This Incan grain-like food, integral to agriculture in the Andes region of South America, has finally made it big in North America. Ok, maybe not *that* big, but it is certainly gaining in popularity—and for good reason. Very few plant foods contain all of the essential amino acids, which are typically only *all* found in animal protein sources. Quinoa (pronounced in the United States as keen-wa, although overseas is pronounced key-no-ah) is packed with fiber, manganese, copper, folate, magnesium, and other nutrients and is low in fat, which makes it a wise addition to any meal. The highlight is really in the quality of the protein it provides, which well exceeds that of almost every other plant (soy is another in this category)—

and there is a lot to be said for that. One of those essential amino acids (essential here means it must come from the diet, since the body can't make it itself) is lysine, essential for tissue growth and repair and a good nutrient to boost your brain health.

When it comes to your waistline, keep the portion size in mind. A full cup of cooked quinoa provides around 220 calories, 4 grams of fat, 39 grams of carbohydrate, 5 grams of fiber, and 8 grams of protein. It makes a nice side dish for fish (or any lean meat), and is also great served at breakfast topped with berries. Quinoa can be found in many mainstream grocery stores these days, so if you have trouble locating it, don't be shy—ask someone to help you.

Go Green

There are many good-for-you green foods out there, but the superfood that often gets overlooked is avocado, a heart-healthy fat that is also good for your brain. The potassium content in avocado helps to lower blood pressure, and when coupled with this food's tendency to increase blood flow, avocados truly are a benefit to your brain. Since this is a fat, it helps you to better absorb fat-soluble vitamins like vitamin A and all the related compounds that act as antioxidants. Avocados also have anti-inflammatory properties. But, as with so many foods, portion size does matter. Since this is a fat-containing food the calories still can add up quickly, so watch how much you are eating; you can still get the health benefits without overdoing it. In one-fifth of a medium avocado, which is about 1 ounce, there are roughly 50 calories, 4.5 grams of fat (3.5 grams of which are unsaturated and heart healthy), and 2 grams of fiber. Not sure what to do with an avocado, other than make guacamole? Try it as a topping on a sandwich or salad.

Don't Forget the Seeds

Seeds, just like nuts, are good for your brain; and just like nuts they are also high in the good fats, meaning you shouldn't overdo it on portion size. Three seeds to add to your brain-boosting, weight-dropping diet include:

- **Sunflower seeds:** These contain tryptophan, which the body can convert to serotonin to boost your mood. They also contain magnesium, which helps lower blood pressure and may reduce your risk of stroke. Not interested in eating them raw? You can now find sunflower seed butters at many grocery stores.
- **Pumpkin seeds:** Just like sunflower seeds, these contain tryptophan, which can really help keep you in a good mood and prevent carbohydrate cravings. They also contain phytosterols—compounds that can help to lower cholesterol levels. Any positive effect on your heart will ultimately promote the health of your brain, making these seeds a bonus in your diet.
- **Chia seeds:** You may not have heard of these seeds yet, but they are gaining in popularity for a good reason. They're a great source of omega-3 fatty acids. However, at this time there's no evidence from the research on chia seeds and weight loss to show that these have an effect on appetite or weight loss, or even heart health. Of course, if there is a benefit to your brain, that could be enough to help keep you focused and making healthy choices every day, and *that* is what will help you lose the weight and keep it off.

Are You Nuts?

Just like avocados, nuts are high in the good fats and offer the added benefit of protecting your brain. Nuts also supply you with minerals, fiber, and protein. Plus, as a bonus, nuts also provide the resources your body needs for your brain to produce mood-boosting serotonin. The magnesium content also provides a brain benefit, because this nutrient helps insulate nerve fibers and this helps them fire faster and more efficiently. At the top of the list for keeping your heart healthy and your blood flowing are walnuts, pecans, almonds, and hazelnuts.

All nuts are high in calories per serving because they are filled with good fats, so limit your intake to one ounce (roughly twenty-four almonds) daily in order to keep your weight loss goals on track. Don't forget to aim for unsalted nuts. A one-ounce serving of almonds contains around 160 calories, 14 grams of fat, 3 grams of fiber, and 6 grams of protein. No need to get stuck on one nut. Try a variety: pistachios, walnuts, almonds, pecans, cashews, hazelnuts, Brazil nuts.

Seeds are a great addition to your diet. Not sure if you will like some of the more exotic seeds? Make sure to give them a try. You may be pleasantly surprised!

Make It Whole

Whole grains are a great addition to a healthy diet and provide fiber, which helps in lowering cholesterol and managing weight. But be sure to read the label; if it doesn't say "whole grain" you aren't getting the same benefits. Additionally, a food may have whole grains but could be mixed with refined grains—so look for "100 percent whole grain" on the label and check to make sure the first ingredient is whole grain. Oats and wheat are great whole grains to start with and easy to find. Other great whole grains include barley, corn, millet, rice, buckwheat, bulgur, farro, spelt, and rye. Aim to make half your grain intake each day from whole grain foods. This works out to about three to five servings per day (as a general goal).

A serving is ½ cup cooked brown rice, ½ cup cooked oatmeal, 1 slice of 100 percent whole-grain bread, 1 ounce of uncooked whole-grain pasta, or 1 cup of 100 percent whole-grain cereal. Or, consider it this way: 16 grams of a whole grain counts as one serving. Look for the "whole grains" stamp on foods to make it easy to see how much you are eating. For more information on whole grains, check out: *www.wholegrainscouncil.org*.

Soy Delicious

There are many benefits to having soy as part of your diet. It is low in fat and a great source of protein. Soy has been linked with lowering blood cholesterol levels as well as reducing blood clots, resulting in better cardiovascular health—which, in turn, means better brain health. Soy also enhances the elasticity of arterial walls, allowing for better blood flow. The biggest benefit of eating soy is that it's a low-fat source of complete protein, which is beneficial to health when it is used to replace saturated fats from animal sources of protein. Sources of soy include tofu, edamame (immature, green soy beans), soy milk, mature soybeans, tempeh (fermented soybean cake), and soy-based "dairy" products. You can also find soy in soy sauce and miso (fermented soy paste), but watch out for the sodium content. Soybean oil is another source—but, like all oils, too much can negatively impact weight, so pay attention to how much you are using.

DID SOMEONE SAY CHOCOLATE?

We did! Chocolate is good for both your body *and* brain, but only in moderation. Henriette van Praag and colleagues from the Salk Institute found that a compound in cocoa, known as epicatechin, combined with exercise, promoted functional changes in an area of the brain that plays a role in learning and memory. There is room in a healthy diet for a little chocolate, and fitting some in here and there will help you avoid feeling deprived or like you have to hide from a chocolate craving. A one-ounce square, up to three times a week, is enough to get the benefits for your brain, and also benefits your sweet tooth. The benefit is in the cocoa itself, so stick with dark or even semisweet chocolate. Milk chocolate is not the best choice because it has added ingredients and saturated fat that reduces the benefits that chocolate can provide. Chocolate's benefits include the following:

- It contains tryptophan, the precursor required to make the neurotransmitter serotonin, which boosts your mood and makes you happy. No wonder we crave it when we're feeling down!
- It contains flavonoids that act as antioxidants and help protect your cells.
- It contains an amino acid that assists in dilating your blood vessels, and serves as a natural anti-inflammatory.
- It contains phytochemicals, which help prevent arterial damage.

Food First

With hundreds of supplements on the market it can be tempting to find every marketed fix for what ails you. The only problem is that you just can't be sure about what you are buying and the lack of regulation in the supplement industry (it is not the same as with food) makes it even harder to know for sure. On top of that, you may not get the same benefit from taking a pill that you would from eating those nutrients as part of actual foods. Supplements are just that—a supplement. These aren't a replacement for a healthy diet or nutrient-packed meals. If you feel you need a supplement, check with your doctor first, consider meeting with a registered dietitian, and check with your pharmacist (to make sure it won't interact negatively with any medications you are taking). And always do your research!

Plus, chocolate contains theobromine, caffeine, and other substances that just might boost your concentration and help you find the focus you need to get your habits on board the healthy train and guide your body to its best shape yet.

FEED YOUR BRAIN, FEED YOURSELF, GET THIN

The first place to start for a healthy brain and a healthy body is with the diet. A poor diet will not only promote obesity and malnutrition, but will also prevent you from thinking clearly and making wise decisions, and could even impact how your brain functions while you're at work. When it comes to getting yourself to the weight you desire—your *thin*—you need to pay attention to what, and how much, you are eating.

Getting the right balance of nutrients will help you manage your weight and help you keep your brain functioning at its best. The foods mentioned here are just some of those that work to power your brain, but they can't do the job alone. It's up to you to make the right choices, incorporate these brain-boosting foods, and fill the rest of your diet with nutrient-rich choices that will help keep you feeling satisfied and knowing that you are feeding your body the right way. Being in a better mood will keep you more motivated to keep eating the right foods, and a clear head will help you when you are faced with tough decisions about food.

AFTERWORD

Congratulations! By completing this book you have just taken the first step toward getting your weight under control. Remember, training your brain to get thin is a total lifestyle change and losing weight can't—and won't—happen overnight. Just know that using the tools provided to you in this book will get you started on the right path to reaching your thin weight, and keeping it there.

Understanding your brain and its components helps you to be in control of what you want. Knowing how to exercise your mind in the right way means you can stay in control of your decisions. Meditation, mental rehearsal, and those similar techniques you just learned about will be handy helpers on your quest for thin, but only if you make sure to practice them regularly. In addition, getting the right amount of sleep, balanced with play, physical activity, and a nutritious diet, will help you get to the weight you want with the body you desire, and most importantly, when you continue with these changes as part of your everyday life, you will be able to keep the weight off.

Your brain plays a critical role in all that you do and it's hard to think of a weight loss plan that doesn't include this component and you're now ready to make the right decision to implement these techniques. You're on your way to committing to a lifetime of healthy choices that will all work together to keep your body at a healthy weight for you. What are you waiting for? It's time to get going and train your brain to get thin!

APPENDIX

SPECIFIC THINGS YOU CAN DO TO TRAIN YOUR BRAIN TO GET THIN

This book has provided you with specific techniques for maximizing the potential of your brain. We know that much of the information was on the complex side because there is a lot of science related to your brain and how it works. As a result, we know that a lot of the book required a little bit of extra work to process—which is, of course, also good for your brain.

Having an understanding of how your brain works and how you can capitalize on its power can help you get what you want out of life, but most importantly this will help you get yourself to the weight you want. So let's wrap things up with a list of some specific things you can do, utilizing the techniques you've learned throughout the book that will train your brain to get thin. After going through the book, you may have a better idea about what you can specifically add to your own list that would be even more specific to your own personal situation.

- Gain an understanding of yourself and your core values, so you have a clear direction of where you see yourself headed.
- Determine what being thin really means to you, and determine if this is a realistic weight goal.
- Make yourself familiar with the most up-to-date information in neuroscience, and then implement those techniques that will strengthen your brainpower.

- Identify your brain's assets and flaws, then work to make your brain a finely tuned thought machine.
- Recognize which activities you do that motivate your brain, as well as which activities have a negative effect.
- Avoid situations that could be considered toxic, where you feel like those around you are lowering your ability to succeed.
- Surround yourself with people who are optimistic and supportive of your weight loss plans.
- Set clear intentions and goals, aiming to solicit your brain's assistance in bringing your dreams into reality.
- Enhance your brain's ability to focus intently on important tasks geared at getting your behaviors in line with being healthy.
- Invest the necessary time and energy needed to fully engage your brain and let it be your partner in weight loss.
- Improve your memory of past successes, which will allow your brain to help you recreate them in future situations that are similar, instead of jumping to fear-based reactions with a focus on negative past experiences and failures.
- Use visualization to generate a mental picture that seems real enough for your brain to perceive it as true, thereby taking you down the neuronal path to recreate the event successfully.
- Strengthen your memory and ability to integrate newly learned information and skills.
- Hone your intuitive powers.
- Go out of your way to do things that shake up your traditional thinking patterns.
- Find new ways to stimulate the parts of your brain that usually lay dormant.
- Don't think in black and white.
- Look at every experience from a different angle.
- Put your brain to the test by challenging it, which will help generate new neuronal pathways.

- Never stop learning. Keep your brain alert and ready to acquire new skills.
- Always seek credible information and learn how to integrate that into your lifestyle.
- Select activities that promote positive outcomes and boost serotonin levels.
- Use positive reinforcement, rewarding yourself in healthy ways.
- Quiet an overactive amygdala, putting an end to irrational fears and improving your decision-making skills.
- Decrease your level of stress to avoid flooding your brain with cortisol.
- Harness the power of meditation to teach your brain how to zap distractions and instead allow you to focus on necessary tasks.
- Train your brain to wash away all negative thoughts and allow yourself to respond more readily to all things in a positive manner.
- Create dedicated playtime.
- Get adequate sleep each night so that every morning you face your challenges feeling refreshed.
- Nourish your body by focusing your caloric needs on nutrient-rich foods so you can properly fuel your brain.
- Allow your blood vessels to remain flexible and clear so your brain has proper blood flow to function properly.
- Provide your brain with space to breathe, making sure it is refreshed and ready to work for you when you need to call upon it.

INDEX

C

D

E

F

O

P

Q

R

S

W

ABOUT THE AUTHORS

Melinda Boyd, MPH, MHR, RD, is a registered dietitian who's spent more than seven years practicing in the field. Her main area of focus is weight management and helping people develop healthier lifestyles. She completed her graduate work at the University of Nevada, Las Vegas, and the University of Oklahoma, and is currently working on a doctoral degree. Melinda lives in Japan with her husband and their two pets.

Michele Noonan, PhD, is an expert in the neuroscience of weight loss. She formulates top-selling health and weight loss supplements and, as the editor-in-chief of *www.doctormichele.com*, she shares "Scientifically Proven Tips for Better Living." Dr. Michele has starred as part of the "Brains" team on the hit CBS reality TV show *Big Brother 11* and has lent her neuroscience expertise to other TV and radio shows. She lives in Los Angeles, California.